One Simple Text...

The Liz Marks Story

Betty Shaw *with Dave Brown*

For information, contact
MSI Press
1760-F Airline Highway, #203
Hollister, CA 95023

Cover photo courtesy the St. Michaels Fire Department.

Back cover photo of Dave Brown: Kim Brown.

Permission granted by Oprah Winfrey Network for use of the photo of Betty Shaw, Oprah Winfrey, and Liz Marks after Betty and Liz's appear-ance on Oprah's *Where are They Now?* show in August 2015.

Permission to use photo of Liz and Betty with hosts of *The Doctors* was granted by Edith Walters, CBS Network.

The author thanks Dr. Dorafshar for providing medical photographs of Liz and for granting permission to use them in this book.

A number of the names in this book are pseudonyms to protect the privacy of the individuals involved.

Library of Congress Control Number 2019949874

ISBN: 978-1-933455-51-8

DEDICATION

**To all the victims of distracted driving accidents,
along with their families. Our thoughts and prayers are with you.**

Betty Shaw

CONTENTS

PREFACE

I was in a near death car accident on April 7, 2012.

My face was shattered, and I suffered a traumatic brain injury. I was not expected to live, but by some miracle I did.

My journey to recovery and acceptance of the new me was far more difficult than I imagined.

I questioned why God let me live. Begging Him to let me die, I went into a deep depression.

I had more than 16 operations to repair the damage caused to my face, ears, and eyes.

I felt left out and lonely because I lost my friends on my way to recovery.

This all happened to me because I chose to text and drive.

This is my story.

Liz Marks

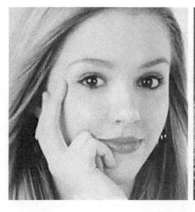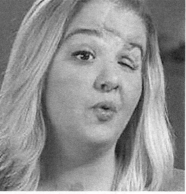

Betty Shaw

ACKNOWLEDGEMENTS

Betty Shaw:

I wish to thank my co-author, Dave Brown. This book would never have made it to print were it not for Dave's knowledge and dedication. I am truly grateful to Dave for his patience, guidance, and friendship throughout the process.

I would also like to thank the St. Michaels Fire Department volunteers, Talbot County Department of Emergency Services community, and the devoted employees of R. Adams Cowley Shock Trauma Center, Kennedy Krieger Institute, and Johns Hopkins Hospital. Thanks to all of you for choosing a career that saves lives.

Next to thank is Dr. Amir H. Dorafshar for use of his photos and encouragement that he provided me over the years not to give up on the book. Thanks also to Lori Millen, Clay Stamp, and MIEMSS for their key roles in helping my daughter bring her story to the masses. Their desire to help Liz will never be forgotten and forever will be appreciated. A special thanks, as well, to Liz's ocularist, Mr. Friel, for his amazing talent in giving Liz two beautiful eyes.

Finally, I would like to extend a heartfelt thanks to my family:
- To my husband for putting up with all my long nights in front of the computer and never once complaining. "Thank you, honey."

- To my children, Logan and Liz. You are the treasures of my soul, and I know your sister Julie is watching over you.

Dave Brown:

First, I would like to thank Betty Shaw. It was an honor to collaborate with her on a book about Liz's incredible journey. I appreciate that Betty asked me to participate. Thank you also to my family, especially my wife Kim for her undying patience and support.

Betty Shaw and Dave Brown:

We would like to thank Betty Lou Leaver of MSI Press for believing in our book and for her tireless work throughout the project, Carl Leaver, also of MSI Press, for his great work on the design of the front and back covers, as well as the book's photo section and typesetting of the book.

Additionally, we want to thank Emma Copley Eisenberg for her editorial excellence, Trudy Stafford for her careful review of the manuscript, and Elizabeth Downey for her kind assistance with the photo section.

Part One

TRAGEDY

"We don't even know how strong we are until we are forced to bring that hidden strength forward. In times of tragedy, of war, of necessity, people do amazing things. The human capacity for survival and renewal is awesome."
Isabel Allende

CHAPTER 1
SATURDAY, APRIL 7, 2012

The morning before Easter I stood in front of the kitchen window in my pajamas with a cup of hot coffee in my hand, gazing at the cloudless sky and watching the pesky squirrels in the backyard eat all of the birdseed out of the birdfeeder. No matter how many times I chased them off, they came back. I loved watching the birds so I put up with the thieves. Such a perfect day—except for one thing: my daughter Elizabeth still wasn't home.

She had spent the night at a friend's house, and I had expected her to return before now. She knew the rules—she had to check in with us in person the next morning after staying the night away from home—but she hated to follow them. A typical teenager, rebellious and stubborn, she thought her parents didn't understand her, that we had no idea what it was like to be a teenager.

Lord knows, I was well aware of the trouble a teenager could get into by spending the night away from home, not only from her older half-brother Logan but also from being a young foolish teenager myself. I sometimes picked up her clothes, smelling for that all-too-familiar, illegal aroma, or leaned in casually to smell her breath for lingering traces of alcohol.

At 10:45, I finally pulled myself away from the window and started to make breakfast, for my husband, Jim, and me: eggs sunny side up. The cooking made me anticipate with more than a little pleasure the annual Easter holiday get-together at our house, a lift I sorely needed after losing my father just a few months prior to colon cancer and then coming face-to-face with my 50th birthday.

Just then, my cell phone beeped with a text message. In 2012, texting was fairly new but had quickly become the norm. Everyone, from teenagers to parents, had a cell phone. Texting was quick, easy and convenient—with no backtalk from your teenager—but could be dangerous if used while driving. The local paper overflowed with stories about the rise in car accidents due to distracted teenage drivers so I made sure that Elizabeth never used her phone when she was driving. She knew the risks and assured me she would never so stupidly use her phone behind the wheel.

The beep signaled a text from Elizabeth about running late for work at a pizzeria where she cut slices for college tuition and spare change and therefore could not check in at home. A bolt of angry disappointment raced through me—she knew the rules and was breaking them once again. We'd been arguing about things like this a lot lately, and I missed our sunnier years less marred by conflict.

"OK," I texted back. Nothing more. No "I love you" like we normally ended our text messages. I wanted her to feel my frustration. Figuring she had already arrived at work, I told myself that I would confront her later when she got home. I waited for her to text me back "I love you" to clear the air, but she never did.

I put the frying pan on the stove, turned on the burner, and sprayed the pan with oil. While the frying pan warmed, I reached into the refrigerator for the egg carton and felt a wave of dizziness and nausea wash over me. I grabbed the counter to keep from falling; it felt like the wind had been knocked out of me. Jim walked into the kitchen at that moment, and I told him that I felt sick to my stomach.

"Really, what brought that on?" he asked.

"I don't know," I said, "but I am going to lie down."

In our bedroom, I covered my head with the blanket to block out the sunlight, which was making my head pound. Soon, I drifted off to sleep.

I don't know how long I slept, only that the sound of our front doorbell startled me awake. I heard my husband's footsteps heading toward the front door, but after that I could not make out anything—just a voice, mumbling, and then the sound of someone running down the hallway toward the bedroom. Pulling the covers off my head, I saw Jim's body filling the doorway and instinctively riveted my eyes on his ashen face. His skyblue eyes, suddenly saucer-sized, dripped tears.

"Who is it?" I screamed. "Who is it?"

In a soft, whimpering voice, he replied, "It's Elizabeth."

I remember running down the hallway, no longer inside my body but rather outside it. I watched myself run and stumble to the front door. I watched myself turn the corner and see a Maryland state trooper standing in the doorway. I stopped in a void of total silence, a kind of silence I had never experienced before. Then, a huge gust of air pushed me back into my body, and I began to tremble.

The state trooper held a walkie-talkie close to his mouth. I have no memory of what he looked like, but I remember he had on a big brown hat and a tan uniform. When he saw me, he stopped talking and looked straight into my eyes.

"Is she alive?! Is she alive?!" I shouted at him.

"Yes," he said, and for a moment I felt relief. Then, he added, "But it doesn't look good."

He bowed his head so all I saw was the top of that big, brown, wide-brimmed hat. The bowing of his head said it all.

"My life is over," I screamed. Then I screamed it again. I raised my arms into the air. I felt a heavy weight pressing down on me. I could not breathe.

Jim put his arms around me, and I calmed down enough to hear what the state trooper had to say. He wanted me to sit down on our couch, but I resisted. I wanted to yell and lose control. I hit my husband a few times in his chest. He grabbed my arms and forced me to sit down on the couch. He sat next to me, as close as he could, and pulled me in so tightly I couldn't move. His body was shaking, but he told me to be still and calm so the officer could speak.

The trooper spoke, but I couldn't listen. He spoke some more. Then, Jim stood up, walked with the officer to the door, and thanked him. I heard the sound of our front door closing. *I cannot believe this is happening*, I thought. *I am only having a nightmare.*

Jim turned to face me again. Our eyes met, but we said nothing. I stood up, headed toward the kitchen, and Jim followed me. I walked to the breakfast bar and stood there. Jim stood on the other side of the bar. We spoke no words, just stood in the kitchen in silence. I thought to myself, *why am I not on my knees praying to God to save my daughter's life? Why am I not running to the car so I can get to her? Why am I not calling my ex-husband—Elizabeth's father—to tell him his daughter is dying?*

I saw myself in the past, and Elizabeth, too. I saw myself pregnant with Elizabeth and her identical twin sister, Julie. Julie had passed away in my womb at 30 weeks of gestation. Elizabeth's father, my ex, and I had already lost one daughter, and now we would have to go through the sorrow of loss again.

Chapter 2

TWINS

I met Logan, son of Frank, the man who would become my husband and Elizabeth's father, in November 1987 when Logan had just turned eight and I, 28, ready to take over raising him. He had short, dark brown, wavy hair, beautiful, straight teeth that gleamed in the light, and olive skin like that of Gail, his mother. The knees of Logan's pants were always covered in mud, and the fridge never stayed full for long when he was around. He and his father shared a passion for crabbing and working on craft projects. I saw this little boy fulfilling my maternal needs.

Logan's father and I married in 1991, and I naively anticipated a Leave-It-to-Beaver ready-made family! Assuming that Logan would accept me right off the bat as his second mom, I felt no need for a child of my own flesh. Mothering Logan would provide the range of emotions that mothers experience—though I idealized those, too. Unfortunately, those unrealistic expectations stressed our marriage from the very start.

Further crumbling the idealized world I had imagined, "stepmother syndrome" soon invaded our relationship. I coveted the intimacy that Logan and his father shared. As for our relationship, Logan had a mother already and didn't want another. He called me Betty. We seemed more like brother and big sister, and we fought like siblings. The battle between the two of us for Frank's attention became a constant tug-of-war. I easily lost patience with Logan and didn't understand how painful it had been for him when his parents divorced and his father remarried. Yet, as the years went by, I learned to protect and care for him as my own child.

Logan wanted badly to have a sister or brother. Early on in our relationship, Logan's father and I decided just having Logan in our lives made us happy, but in my early 30s, those maternal pangs really started to ping. It took some persuasion, but when I turned 32, Frank agreed that we would try to get pregnant. We did not tell Logan we were trying, though, for fear I would not conceive. (In the 1990s—considered by some to be the "old days"—the average age of conception was 24 and many doctors assumed that women at age 30 and beyond would have difficulty conceiving and be at risk for complications to themselves and to their babies though nowadays that age is generally pegged at 35.)

I got off the pill and quickly became pregnant. So much for that worry! I felt too excited to wait the standard three months before telling people about the pregnancy. I was thrilled, not only for me and Frank but also for Logan who so badly wanted a connection with a younger sibling. Being a child of divorced parents can be a lonely experience, and Logan felt we would be more of a real family if he had a sister or brother.

Almost immediately, though, complications dogged this pregnancy. In my eighth week, common smells began to make me horribly nauseous. Whenever I walked into a public restroom, the chemical cleaning odors made my stomach churn. Going out anywhere became a challenge. Finally, I developed the skill of running to the toilet, washing my hands, and reapplying my lipstick, all in less than 60 seconds and while still holding my breath to avoid public restroom smells that made me sick to my stomach. As the weeks wore on, I started to feel queasy day and night. I did not have morning sickness—I had all-day sickness. The only thing I could eat and hold down was a Whopper from Burger King—the only food that did not torture me. Oh, I couldn't get enough of those huge, messy burgers! To them alone, I attributed the extra pounds I put on very early in my pregnancy.

Then, in my fourth month, my obstetrician, Dr. Chang, called with alarming results from blood work done a few days earlier. This blood work should have been done weeks before, but I had procrastinated. Because of the late testing, Dr. Chang attributed the disturbing results to one of three things:

1) The baby could have Down syndrome, which due to my age, 33, was considered a real possibility.

2) I could have a multiple pregnancy.

3) The test had been misread.

Dr. Chang advised me to come into her office the next day for a sonogram that would reveal the answer.

The following day, I drove myself to the appointment. Frank had to work. Unconcerned, he shrugged off any dire expectations. "Don't worry," he reassured me. "Most likely, someone misread the test. Relax. Do what the doctor says, and I'll see you this evening."

So, off I went, not completely reassured. I really wished he could have come. I wished that even more as I lay on the table, watching the technician lube my belly.

"Whoa, there are two!" he exclaimed as he touched the cold wand to my stomach.

I turned my head to look at the screen, but I couldn't see what he saw. He showed me, by outlining with his finger: two small babies so close together they seemed like one.

"Are they okay?" I asked.

A few heart-pounding moments passed.

"Everything looks good," he said. "One baby is smaller than the other, but that's nothing to be too concerned about. Even the smaller baby is within the normal growth rate."

I let out my breath.

"Do you want to know the sex of the babies?" he asked.

"I do."

"You are having twin girls."

"Twins," I repeated. "Are they identical?"

"They are! But so far, I can't tell if they share the same amniotic sac or placenta. It looks like there is a dividing membrane on the sonogram here, but it's too faint to confirm."

I learned that in medical terms, the girls could be monochromic-diamniotic twins, meaning they shared the same placenta but had their own amniotic sac, or they could be monochromic-monoamniotic twins, meaning they shared everything.

Returning home, I sat down at the kitchen table. The shock of learning two babies were growing inside me gave way to relief and joy. I didn't move. I didn't call anyone. I just wanted to tell Frank and have him be the first to know. Logan would be at school and then at a friend's house; Frank and I would tell him together.

Frank ambled through the front door at 5:30 that evening. He looked at me expectantly, and the news just burst out from me. "We're having twins—healthy twins!"

"Oh. Oh?" He seemed agitated rather than pleased.

I felt stung; I thought he would at least be happy that the babies were healthy. I had not contemplated that something might go wrong with the pregnancy or that having a second baby would be even more expensive, but Frank's face suddenly brought all these possibilities home to me.

Frank opened the refrigerator, grabbed a beer, popped open the tab, and heavily took a seat at the table next to me. After a few sips of his beer, he looked at me and asked, "Boys or girls?"

"Girls."

There, finally, appeared the big, joyous smile I'd been looking for. "Let's tell Logan," he said.

When we told Logan, his eyes grew nearly as wide as his smile. "Cool!" he said. "I will have *two* sisters to play with!" Then he added with a wicked grin, "and to mess with!"

In the following months, we fussed and prepared. Such happy times! We decided to name the babies Sara Trudy Marks and Julie Dorothy Marks, middle names after our mothers' first names just because we liked them. We started to refer to them as "the girls."

I bought matching outfits for them, and we saved money to buy the best double stroller available. A contractor by trade, Frank took on extra projects. The age difference between Logan and his soon-to-be sisters matched the age difference between Frank and his sister, Lisa. They enjoyed a very close relationship, and I hoped that Logan and the girls would, too.

Finally, over my morning sickness, I could now enjoy my job as a bank teller better—able to interact with customers without having to block thoughts of the nausea churning in my stomach and to listen longer and without physical distractions to the more experienced mothers who worked with me: their motherhood stories—both the great stuff and the nightmares, their advice on raising a teenage boy, and so much more. A low-key job with supportive co-workers—the right place and the right people at that time! Equally wonderfully, I could eat food other than Whoppers! After all, sometimes those little things count more than the big things!

In the 28th week of my pregnancy, the date of the next sonogram arrived, and this time Frank came along. He wanted to see the girls himself. As for me, I wanted to see how much the girls had grown.

The same friendly technician who'd exclaimed "Whoa, it's twins!" at my first sonogram greeted us. Once again, he lubed my belly. Then, he turned out the light and moved the freezing wand over it. Through the darkness, Frank peered into the screen. In those days, sophisticated 3D imaging had not yet been developed. Still not very detailed, sonograms confused the untrained eye.

I expected the technician's usual informative banter, but this time his mouth twitched and his eyes looked serious. He kept moving the wand around the left side of my belly with intense focus. He slid the wand to the right side of my belly for a quick picture of the other baby and then pushed it back to the left side again. He remained in that spot, taking more and more images of the left-sided baby.

"Is something wrong?" I asked.

"The doctor will answer all of your questions," he said too briefly and without emotion. Then, he turned off the sonogram machine, handed us two pictures—one of each girl—and flipped on the lights.

I sat up and looked at Frank. I could see the fear in his eyes, too. We looked at the pictures, trying to figure out which baby might be in trouble, but we couldn't see any difference between the two images that might indicate danger. We looked at those pictures a long time.

"I can't see anything," Frank said, and I agreed. Then, the door opened. The technician told us to follow him upstairs. Dr. Chang wanted to speak to us.

Dr. Chang, petite, with glasses and short, dark hair cut in a bob, greeted us, telling us to take a seat, and then sat down behind a desk that nearly overwhelmed her, if not in size then in the scores of folders scattered across the top. Usually cool and professional, distant even, this time she spoke slowly and warmly. Without any preamble, she stated that Baby B had a problem and started to provide details.

Confused by the labels, let alone by the situation facing us, Frank stopped her. "Which baby are you talking about" he asked. "The one on the left side or the one on the right side?

"Have you named the babies yet?" she asked.

"Yes," I spoke up, "Sara and Julie."

"Okay, then," Dr. Chang dove right into the essence of the problem, "Baby B, Julie, on your left side needs immediate attention." In this way, Dr. Chang assigned the names we used for each baby after that.

"Julie," she continued, "has grown considerably less than Sara, dangerously so. I'm really worried, given the level of danger and the higher risk of complications for multiple births that we have talked about before. I know you probably don't want to hear this--and I really want you to understand that you have done nothing wrong, absolutely nothing wrong--but we need to deliver these babies by Caesarean section as soon as possible."

Frank's face wrinkled in the same way it had when I told him we were having twins.

"But I'm only 28 weeks!" I cried. "No, no. I am not going to go along with taking the babies so early. I want another option."

"In that case, I'd suggest you go see a specialist at Johns Hopkins Hospital in Baltimore," she advised; she did not display any irritation. "I'll call them and let them know about Julie's condition and that you need to be seen right away. Also, you need to be on bed rest for the remainder of the pregnancy. It's very important that you get plenty of rest and eat healthy, not just for your sake but also for the sake of both babies."

That conversation changed my life, definitely my daily life. The following day, I took a leave of absence from my bank teller job and made an appointment at Johns Hopkins. As with other really good hospitals, Johns Hopkins had no immediate openings. With immense disappointment, I made one for the first possible time: one week later.

In the interim, I began using the portable heart monitor Dr. Chang's staff had given me and taught me to use, especially what to listen for. Every 2-3 hours I checked on Julie's heartbeat, listening for any signs of change. Both the monitoring and the wait to get into Johns Hopkins constituted an ongoing emotionally gut-wrenching seven days.

I let Dr. Chang know, and she had me come in every day so that she could check on the girls. Luckily, Julie seemed to be stabilizing—or so I thought, hoped, prayed, and believed.

Finally, the day of the appointment at Johns Hopkins arrived. We arrived, walked through the front door, and stopped—a maze of corridors spread out before us. I worried we would get lost in that maze, but we found the OB/GYN department easily.

Once we had signed in and filled out the proper paperwork, a hospital aide met us. "Please come with me, both of you," he said. "I will take you to the sonogram room."

He led us down another corridor. Never would we have made our own way there!

Like everything we had seen so far at Johns Hopkins, the size of the room impressed us. Both the machine and the room were much larger than the room and sonogram equipment at Dr. Chang's. I liked the pretty, golden-yellow walls and the sunshine flooding through the oversized windows. That golden aura had a much-needed calming effect on me.

After a few short minutes, our new OB/GYN doctor entered the room. She had long, light brown hair, and under a white doctor's coat, a thin frame. She introduced herself confidently as Dr. Valerie Kelvin, smiled, and shook our hands.

Johns Hopkins is a teaching hospital so at least four other people in the room observed as Dr. Kelvin administered the sonogram. This sonogram took a long time—Dr. Kelvin was being extremely thorough. Though Johns Hopkins had more current sonogram technology, Frank and I could still make out next to nothing when we looked at the screen.

"I've seen worse," Dr. Kelvin said.

I let out the breath I'd been holding. Frank smiled widely.

We knew that Dr. Kelvin had received Dr. Chang's notes and sonogram images of the girls so those words reassured us beyond perhaps what they should have. Dr. Kelvin then informed us that she had a meeting, but that she and other doctors would meet with us in 90 minutes to go over their suggested plan of action. Then, she called over a tall young man in blue scrubs and introduced him as Dr. Roger O'Donnell.

To put us at ease—and likely also to kill those 90 minutes of waiting time—Dr. O'Donnell showed Frank and me to the Neonatal Intensive Care Unit (NICU), reserved for authorized personnel and parents or guardians, where the girls would be transferred after delivery. He promised to do everything possible to deliver Julie and Sara safely. Then, he ushered us into a conference room where an imposing group of medical professionals sat around a smooth round table. Doctors in white coats sat interspersed with three doctors in training and a woman with a clipboard. Dr. O'Donnell showed us to our seats and sat down next to me. He offered quick introductions, and then the meeting began.

The doctors lobbed medical terms at each other while Frank and I sat in the stands like the estranged parents of a tennis star watching the sport for the first time—we cared about the outcome but had no idea what the plays meant. After a few minutes, Dr. Kelvin turned to us.

"It's still unclear if the girls share the same amniotic sac or not. They do share the same placenta, which makes not knowing if they also share the same sac a big concern. If they share the same amniotic sac and Julie expires in the womb, then Sara will soon expire as well." Frank reached out and took my hand at that word, *expire*, spoken frighteningly matter-of-factly.

"The girls look to be at 30 weeks' gestation [Waiting for the appointment had given them a little more time!] so their lungs are not fully developed," Dr. Kelvin continued. "Delivering the babies that early would be a big risk. I recommend giving each girl a steroid shot to promote the growth of her lungs. Hopefully within a week or two, depending on how much the lungs grow and how well Julie holds up, we would deliver the girls via C-section, then rush them to the NICU. But I must warn you, steroid shots can terminate one or both of the pregnancies."

The plan: I would stay in the hospital overnight so the doctors could monitor the girls. Once home, I'd have daily visits with Dr. Chang, who would maintain contact with Dr. Kelvin until the day of my scheduled C-section.

That night in the hospital, every time I started to drift off to sleep, a nurse would come in saying sorry, but she had to check the girls' heart-beats. I watched her facial expressions for any signs of trouble. The last checkup was 6:00 a.m. The nurse said everything sounded good and went to take care of other patients. At 9:00, one of the interns wheeled me out of my room and took me for one last sonogram before I could go home. He joked about the hospital food and smells, and I laughed and laughed, as much from nervousness as levity.

Once in the small nook of a sonogram room, I felt the familiar cold lubrication of the sonogram wand on my belly. The intern continued to chat with me as he worked. I was answering a question when he interrupted me and said firmly, "Please be quiet."

How rude, I thought. Then I saw his face—the same panicked expression as the technician who'd made the first discovery about Julie. Once again that wand lingered too long on my left side.

"I'll be right back," he said in a rushed voice.

Suddenly, someone ripped the curtain around my bed aside so hard that part of it came down from its hanger. It was Dr. Kelvin. She grabbed the sonogram wand and went directly to the left side of my belly.

"I am sorry to tell you this," she said, pushing the sonogram machine aside, "but Baby B has no heartbeat. We are taking you to get an emergency C-section now."

Four people in blue scrubs hurried into the room, each grabbed a corner of my bed, and off we sailed down the hallway. I remember the ceiling and how fast the lights passed me overhead. The sonogram room was in a distant area of the hospital so they had to get me to the main hospital operating rooms. Stat!

Arriving breathlessly in the operating room, one of the attendants deftly gave me a spinal block. After that, I felt no pain, only pressure. I could not see anything, either, because a big plastic sheet separated me from my stomach and from the doctors, who talked in slow bursts of sound. I tried to listen to the doctors' words, but an anesthesiologist kept firing irrelevant questions at me—distracting me, I realized later.

Finally, I heard a baby crying—and then I saw Baby A, Sara. Her face, the only part of her visible from behind the nurse's white cloth, was horribly bruised black and blue. The nurse brought her to me.

"Not to worry," the nurse said. "She isn't in pain; she's just been positioned at the bottom of your stomach. It was your legs moving during the pregnancy that bruised her like that."

"Did we make it in time to save Julie?" I asked.

"We're working on her."

I prayed to God that we had made it in time.

They took me into a recovery room, cleaned me up, and hooked me up to machines. I felt some pain—contractions, I was later told—so they medicated me. I can't tell you the exact moment when everything happened, only that one baby was born alive and the other wasn't.

I lay there in the room for a while, wondering, alone. Then, Dr. Kelvin came in.

"Betty," she said. "Baby A was born safely and is doing well. She weighed in at three pounds six ounces. She is stable and is being examined in the NICU unit." I waited. "I'm sorry, but Baby B didn't make it." She paused again. "Do you want to see her?"

"No," I said. I felt so alone. Frank had gone home the night before to drop Logan off at Lisa's and to take care of any work issues he had. He had planned to return in the morning to take me home. Before cell phones, instant communication did not occur, but the nurse had managed to get a call through so he was now aware and on his way. It would take him 45 minutes, though—45 minutes when I was on my own, responsible for making decisions no one should have to make, and feeling lost, bereft, and, of course, confused and even, rightly in my mind, somewhat angry at no one, everyone, all of life.

Dr. Kelvin was replaced by a nurse in her early 20s, slightly overweight, with a pretty face. She came up to me.

"Why don't you want to see your baby?"

How dare you, I thought. *You have no idea what I've been through.*

But then, she took my hand firmly. "I had a baby that I lost at birth not long ago," she said, in a voice shot through with real empathy and much older than her years. "Don't be disconnected from your daughter," she said.

"This is your one and only time to tell her you love her and say goodbye." She asked if she could please bring the baby in for me to hold.

"Yes."

She returned with Julie.

"Hi, everyone," she said to those bustling around the busy recovery room. "Can we give Betty a moment alone with her child?"

They finished their tasks and left. She placed Julie in my arms. Julie was wrapped up in a white blanket just like her sister. Her face was not bruised like Sara's. She was so small—her arm only the width of a pencil.

"What's her name?" the nurse asked.

"Julie," I said, my voice breaking.

I loosened the blanket, pulled out her hand, which was still warm, and held it.

"Kiss her hand," the nurse said. "Breathe in her scent all the way until it reaches your soul. Talk to your daughter as if she were alive. Tell her how much you love her and how much she will be missed in your life."

I did as she told me. I will never forget that nurse. I will forever hold those moments with my daughter Julie within me. April 22, 1994 was the date of Julie's death and Sara's birth.

~~~~~~~~~~~~~~~

In the weeks that followed, Baby A thrived, and Frank and I decided to rename her. Without Julie, the name "Sara" simply didn't make sense—it had always been Julie and Sara, our girls. Frank suggested that we name Baby A after me—he had always liked that my older sister was named after our mother. My legal name is Elizabeth, though I have always been called Betty. We decided to call Baby A Elizabeth.

CHAPTER 3
GETTING TO ELIZABETH

I careened around Elizabeth's room, looking for something, anything, that felt like her that I could hold onto. Then, I saw it: her pillow—her favorite, the one she slept on every night, the one with the pizza stains, blotches of makeup, and the fruity scent of her perfume. I clutched that pillow to my chest for the whole ride to Shock Trauma in Baltimore. The drive had taken more than an hour, a span that people tend to think must have felt like an eternity. But it didn't. I wanted that drive to last forever. I feared that once we arrived at Shock Trauma, they would tell us Elizabeth was dead. As long as the car rolled along the road, Elizabeth was alive.

Paramedics had flown Elizabeth in a medevac helicopter from a cleared crop field a half-mile from the accident scene to the roof of the R. Adams Cowley Shock Trauma Center, part of the University of Maryland Medical Center—Shock Trauma for short. There, she'd been rushed to the emergency room. The center had been named for Dr. Cowley, "the father of trauma medicine" and the man who coined the term "golden hour" believing it critical for a patient who had sustained a brain injury to receive medical treatment within an hour lest the injury be fatal.

I grabbed the first clothing I saw and the Bible that I've had since I was a little girl and that holds a few strands of my father's grey hair. By the grace of God, Frank had been working just a few miles away on a contracting job when I called and told him the news. He appeared at our door within five minutes.

My husband drove. As we made our first turn out of our neighborhood, I heard words being spoken to me from inside my body: "She will be okay; it is happening for a reason." I felt them again, "She will be okay; it is happening for a reason." I turned to Frank, who was sitting in the back seat and held out my hand. He took it. Together, we cried.

We had nearly reached the hospital when my cell phone rang with the number of Shock Trauma.

"Are you Elizabeth Marks's mother?"

"Yes!"

"This is Doctor Sutcliffe. We have your daughter here at Shock Trauma," he said. "Does your daughter have any medical conditions that could affect her treatment?"

"No, none." Then I screamed into the phone, "You have my consent to do whatever it takes to save my daughter's life!"

"I'll do the best I can. How far away are you?"

"Twenty minutes."

"Hurry," he said.

When we reached Shock Trauma, Jim dropped Frank and me off at the main entrance of the hospital not at the rather distant Shock Trauma Building of the University of Maryland Medical Center. Dodging people, we sprinted straight to the front desk. Though a crowd of people had gathered in line waiting to be helped, the woman behind the desk must have seen the fear in my eyes because she stopped talking to the person in front of her and asked us, "Who are you here for?"

She got on her computer, then picked up the phone, and after a few moments told us that someone was coming. I saw a young woman with a hospital badge draped around her neck running toward us.

"Are you Elizabeth Marks's parents?"

"Yes!"

"Follow me."

We ran through the hospital, weaving left and right around circles of people until we came to an elevator. When the doors closed, she inserted a key into the floor button panel and pushed 4. The sound when we stepped out of the elevator deafened me. I turned to my left and saw a thick team of doctors and nurses working on someone lying on a bed. It was not until our escort pointed it out that I realized the person at the center of all this noise and emergency labor was Elizabeth.

I stood stock still outside the action, watching doctors and nurses lean over the bed, then rush back to get something only to return to the bed again. I heard them yelling commands to each other and unwrapping equipment from paper casings. Jim appeared by my side, and the three of us, Jim, Frank, and I, just stood there in shock. Jim started sobbing. Then, Frank did, too, his shoulders slumped like a man defeated. But no tears came for me. I just stood there, stoic.

At that point, Dr. Sutcliffe took me aside, telling me, "Elizabeth is holding her own."

I couldn't believe it—she was not dead yet! I had made it! I would have the chance to say goodbye before she died!

The words Dr. Sutcliffe said next have etched themselves indelibly into my memory: "Mrs. Shaw, on a scale of one to four, four being the worst, we are grading your daughter over three."

Over three!! I didn't care how bad she was, I would take her in any condition. Just keep her alive! *God, you already took Julie from me*, I begged, *please don't take Elizabeth, too.*

"She's going to need emergency surgery," Dr. Sutcliffe continued. "Many procedures."

I pushed through the many white-coated and blue-uniformed bodies. I went right up to her face, which had sustained visually obvious damage, but nothing stopped me, her mother after all, from speaking to that face, to my beloved daughter.

"Don't leave earth," I whispered to her, the words bursting from my very soul. "Stay here with Daddy and me. You are the joy of my life. I love you."

Not allowed to touch Elizabeth because of the need to keep everything sterile, I folded my hands in prayer and got as close to Elizabeth as possible. I repeated those words over and over and over. "Stay with us...please...I love you." No tears ran down my face. All my emotions had frozen in shock, desperation, fear, and primal love. Outward calm belied inner turmoil, inexpressible in its depth.

After too short a time, Dr. Sutcliffe firmly grasped my arm and maneuvered me into a quiet space to update Frank, Jim, and me on Elizabeth's condition and his plan of action. The plan included a quick CT scan. That scan would dictate the next steps to be taken. Then, Dr. Sutcliffe and two blue-uniformed interns rolled Elizabeth out of the room.

The three of us—Frank, Jim, and I—had been standing together, alone, not talking, not knowing what to say, outside the cubicle that had housed Elizabeth for barely three minutes when the interns brought the gurney with my daughter back. Dr. Sutcliffe followed right behind them—with frightening news. "No time to wait," he stated curtly. "We need to operate right now."

After Frank and I had quickly signed surgical consent papers, Dr. Sutcliffe advised us, "The operation will take 4-5 hours. If your daughter survives, you can see her after that."

I remember watching someone shave Elizabeth's long, beautiful, blonde tresses, of which she was very proud, in preparation for surgery. How strange it felt to see the bundles of blonde fall to the floor. I ran up to the intern shaving Elizabeth's head. "Can I have some of her hair?" I asked.

"We will get you clean hair later," he said, annoyed. "This hair has blood on it."

"No, I want her hair now!" I screamed back.

He turned to look at a nurse who was standing near him, and I heard her say, "Goddam it, give her some of her daughter's hair!" She understood what I was asking for—a piece of Elizabeth while she was still alive.

Then, they took her away. We said our goodbyes quickly, and Dr. Sutcliffe and the group of people keeping Elizabeth alive wheeled her away. One of them pushed a button on the wall, opening the double doors, and Frank, Jim, and I watched as the doors closed.

Right at that point, a chaplain approached me. I was crying now but able to talk.

"Why are you here?" I asked him. Looking surprised, he told me that he'd received a call that his services might be needed. We stood in the space where Elizabeth had just had her hair shorn, and I asked him if we could pray. I bowed my head. As he was saying a prayer for our daughter, my mind flooded with questions about the significance of Dr. Sutcliffe's "over three" rating. Will Elizabeth be a vegetable? Will she know who I am? Is it fair to keep her alive just for me?

When I opened my eyes, I saw drops of Elizabeth's blood on the floor. Then, I looked over and saw the trash can with my daughter's once beautiful long blonde hair hanging out of it.

After my brief talk with the chaplain, Jim and Frank thanked him for his prayer for Elizabeth, as did I. Just then, an aide showed up to direct the three of us to a waiting room just outside the trauma area. I looked down at my right hand. I had not realized that I'd been clenching it tightly—and now it started to hurt. I slowly stretched my fingers to ease the tension. As my fingers started to relax, my eyes focused on what I had been so passionately holding: safely secured in the palm of my hand were the strands of Elizabeth's hair. I opened my Bible, which I had jammed into my purse, and put Elizabeth's hair in the Ziploc bag with my father's treasured hair that I had laid inside that Bible so many months ago. Then, I rubbed the hairs together so they might intertwine. —hairs of the most loved people in my life. I silently and desperately prayed to my dad to please save his granddaughter.

"Don't let God take her away," I pleaded.

CHAPTER 4
AGONIZING WAIT

The waiting room at Shock Trauma filled with family members and Elizabeth's friends. We come from a small town so news of Elizabeth's accident had gotten around quickly. My mom and my sister, Trudy, took me into their arms. I wondered how they'd even known to come. I had no memory of calling them although I had.

My ex-sister-in-law, Lisa, sat with me. "Has anyone called Logan yet?" I asked her.

Even though Frank and I had divorced several years earlier, Logan and I remained close. I worried about how Logan would react to such devastating news about his little sister.

"He booked the first flight to Baltimore," Lisa said.

As Frank and Jim hugged our friends and family and thanked them for coming to be with us at this terrible time, I pulled Trudy aside.

"Take a walk with me?" I asked her, and she agreed.

Sunlight streamed through the big windows that lined the long hallway as we walked. After a time, I stopped walking.

"I may need your help," I said.

"Anything. What is it?"

"The doctors are not hopeful that Elizabeth will make it through her surgery," I began. "If she doesn't make it, I'm not sure how I will react. I'm afraid I'll lose control and won't be able to make good decisions. Do we want to donate Elizabeth's organs? I'm not sure. Her father is in no condition to make that decision, either."

Trudy nodded.

"I need you to be my backup just in case," I continued. "I want to make sure Elizabeth's organs get donated—she would have wanted that." At least, I thought she would have, but I didn't know for certain. She had never told me her wishes, and I had never asked. No parent ever wants to think about that question, let alone speak the words.

Tears ran down Trudy's face. "I promise to be your voice," she said. We stepped closer and hugged a long time in silence.

Next, I asked Jim to walk with me. I was still calm—and numb.

"I'm sorry," I began.

"Sorry for what?"

A 42-year-old bachelor when we married, Jim had no children of his own, and he did not wish to have any. But he cared for Elizabeth and knew she was part of the package.

"If Elizabeth dies," I said, "I will go crazy for a while, but I will come back to you. I won't leave you physically, but mentally I will be gone for a while. Please hang in there, and don't leave me. Give me time to get back to my old self."

I knew that if Elizabeth passed away, I would struggle terribly with life. I had already lost her twin sister, Julie. If I lost Elizabeth as well, life would become colorless, and I would feel like a failure as a mother. How could I let two children die under my care? What did I do wrong as a mom or as a woman to have this happen to me?

"Alcoholism runs in my family," I said, "and I'm afraid I'll use that. I'll just be so sad to miss out on so much with her. I'll never get to be a grandmother to Elizabeth's kids."

Jim hugged me. He said he understood and added, "I am not going anywhere."

I needed to get away from all the attention so Jim took me to an area where his sister, Colleen, and his brother-in-law, Brett, were sitting near a Coffee Shop Hut. I looked at the people standing in line, waiting to place their orders, and wondered who each person was there for and what tragedy might be happening to each of them. It had been exactly an hour and a half since they took Elizabeth into surgery.

As I sat there with these thoughts swirling, a cry went up, directed toward me. "The doctor is looking for you!"

Dr. Sutcliffe had said that the operation would take 4-5 hours unless she didn't make it. I ran to the waiting area, and when I reached it, I saw that all the people there had their eyes on me.

"Where is the doctor?!" I screamed. "Where is Frank?!"

Someone led me to a door and opened it for me. In a small room sat Frank, Lisa, and a number of others, packed like sardines. "What happened?" I screamed. "Is she alive?!"

Then, I heard people telling me to be calm, the news was good. Until that point, I'd tried to stay unemotional, but when I heard those words, something broke inside me. I fell into my sister Debbie's arms, sobbing, and the room fell silent.

I looked at Dr. Aaron, the surgeon who had performed Elizabeth's emergency surgery.

"Elizabeth is one lucky girl," he said. "Her brain injury was not as bad as we thought. Her face took most of the impact, which saved her brain. While she suffered a traumatic brain injury, there was still brain activity. The precise damage will be determined in the days to come after the swelling of her brain goes down. We are not out of the woods—she is still in critical condition. She will be evaluated by other specialists to determine the extent of her other injuries."

We all cried, held each other, and gave Dr. Aaron hugs before he left. As he opened the door, I saw one of Elizabeth's friends standing near the doorway. I gave her a thumbs up, and she ran to tell everyone the good news: "She's alive!"

Betty Shaw

CHAPTER 5

STAYING ALIVE

Walking out of the small room and taking my first deep breath in what seemed like ages, I ran into Tracy, a co-worker of Jim's. A volunteer fire fighter, he had come to the hospital to support Jim. Tracy had been at the accident and, having learned details of the subsequent investigation, informed us that Elizabeth had been at fault.

"Fortunately," he said, "no one else was killed or injured."

That news brought us great relief, but we still did not know what had caused Elizabeth to drive directly into the back of a tow truck stopped in front of her, waiting to make a left turn. Had she been ill? Distracted? What had been so important? Elizabeth, still unconscious, couldn't tell us.

The questions floated through my mind, but deep down, at the time, I really did not care. All my energy flowed to Elizabeth and focused on the aftermath of what had happened to her.

Logan arrived, and we just held on to each other and cried. It had been hours since the last doctors' update about Elizabeth's condition. Day turned into night, and we moved to a waiting room just outside the hospital's Neuro Trauma Critical Care Unit (CC) for spinal cord and brain injury patients.

Family and friends went home. Only Frank, his girlfriend Susan, Jim, Logan, and I remained. Then, Logan and Susan went, too—to a nearby friend's house to get some rest.

Now only two other people shared the waiting room with us: a couple, holding hands. There was no need to exchange pleasantries with them. I could see in their faces that their lives were exploding, just like mine.

At 3:00 in the morning, we received word about Elizabeth.

"Both her eyes were severely damaged," the ophthalmologist told us. "I'm fairly certain that her left eye is damaged beyond repair and that she has lost sight in that eye. Her right eye is too swollen to know for sure, but her retina is still connected. Once the swelling goes down, we will know if she has sight in that eye or not. Other specialists will be coming out with more updates in the coming hours. Any questions?"

We couldn't muster any. He left. The seriousness in his voice sent me down a dark tunnel of thought, asking questions aloud.

"Just be grateful she's still alive," Frank said.

At some point, the other couple from the waiting room left though I don't remember them leaving. The television played instrumental music, the kind you would hear in a dentist's office that is supposed to soothe you and get your mind off the needle. The TV showed pictures over and over of mountains, oceans, and forests. The music and the pictures were supposed to be relaxing. Both Jim and Frank dozed off for a few minutes, but I couldn't. I stood in front of that television with my arms positioned like I was holding a baby and rocking her back and forth.

~~~~~~~~~~~~~~~

Another hour passed. An otolaryngologist came to inform us that he had just examined Elizabeth's ears and they were too swollen for him to provide a definitive assessment on her hearing.

Then, a pulmonologist reported that it was too soon to give us an answer on the condition of Elizabeth's lungs. "She's on life support," he told us. "In critical but stable condition. You may see her now, but only one visitor at a time."

I did not give Frank the chance to go first, I just headed straight for the double doors that would lead me to Elizabeth. My once beautiful, carefree, active girl with long blonde hair was bald. Bandages swaddled her head and eyes. Tubes switch-backed into her head and body. I could not believe that this was my child. She looked so broken.

I listened to the sounds of the machines keeping her alive. In the distance, I heard other patients' machines and listened to their loved ones, talking to them in crying voices. I could not fathom how the people who worked there handled the sadness of the job.

Suddenly I realized a nurse was standing beside me. "Take it hour by hour," she said. "Try not to think too far ahead."

I sat with my Bible in my hand, and I prayed. Then, I let Frank have a turn by Elizabeth's bedside.

Around 5:00 a.m., Frank came back out to the waiting room so that Elizabeth could be examined by the plastics doctor. After 45 minutes or so, the doctor came out.

"Elizabeth sustained major damage to her whole face," he said. "Her nose is broken; her left eye socket is shattered; and her right eye socket has multiple fractures."

I interrupted him. "How bad is her face?"

"One of the worst I have seen," he said. "She will need 20-30 surgeries to repair her face."

The three of us just sat there in disbelief.

~~~~~~~~~~~~~~~

Morning broke. It was Easter Sunday. I called my mom around 7 a.m. to give her the update on Elizabeth. I tried to sound positive, but she knew by my voice the grimness of the situation.

"Please take all the food from my house, and have the gathering at Trudy's house. I know you don't want to, but please do this for me. I want this Easter Sunday to be a celebration that Elizabeth is still alive. Please tell everyone to please say a prayer for Elizabeth and that I love them."

It had been my turn to host the family gathering this year. In spite of everything going on, that weighed on my mind.

My mother was crying, but she agreed to do it. "I'll come to the hospital tomorrow and stay as long as you need me," she said.

When I hung up the phone, I closed my eyes. *Happy Easter, Elizabeth,* I wished in my mind. *Please stay alive.*

Frank, Jim, and I went to the house of a friend who lived nearby, only a few blocks away from Shock Trauma. I didn't want to leave Elizabeth, but both insisted that I get a few hours of sleep and try to eat—I'd had no appetite since the accident. I finally agreed to go with them because the friend lived very close and the hospital staff promised to call if there were any change in Elizabeth's condition.

Susan and Logan were already there. Then, Lisa and her husband Bob arrived. When I saw Lisa, for a brief moment I thought it was Elizabeth standing in front of me and coming in to hug me. She looked so much like Elizabeth. They shared many of the same facial features, and we always joked about how Elizabeth should be her daughter and not mine. I broke down and cried wildly in Lisa's arms.

Then, I regained my composure. "Can everyone gather around to say a prayer?" I asked. We formed a circle and held hands.

I thanked God for not letting anyone else get hurt or killed in the accident. I couldn't imagine what it would be like to have your child take away someone else's loved one, I told God. I asked God to spare her life. I asked God to give us a second chance with her, and I told Him how much we all loved her and needed her in our lives. "Amen."

When I looked up, I saw tears streaming down every face.

In the morning, we returned to Elizabeth's side in CC/ICU. It was time for the others to say their goodbyes to Elizabeth. Frank and Jim were returning to work. Everyone else, too. Logan was flying back to South Carolina but would be keeping in touch every day and had made plans to return in two weeks.

I wouldn't be returning to my current job, Jim and I had decided. I would stay with Elizabeth by day and in a hotel a few blocks from the hospital by night so I could be as close to Elizabeth as possible. Jim would be with me at the hotel each evening when he got off work and would visit with Elizabeth for a while, then make me eat something and go to the hotel for some rest.

Everyone left. I pulled up a chair to get as close to Elizabeth as possible and just stared at her, trying to find parts of this battered young woman lying in the bed in front of me that told me she was my daughter. Sadly, I saw and heard very little besides the noises coming from the machines keeping her alive. She made no sound on her own. Silence.

A nurse came in to check on Elizabeth so I took the opportunity to get a cup of coffee. I wound up at the same coffee shop that I'd noticed when we first arrived at Shock Trauma. Now I was one of those grave people waiting in line.

Back at Elizabeth's bed, I saw one of the nurses who had looked after Elizabeth when she was flown to the Trauma Resuscitation Unit. She saw me and started to clap with excitement, and then she gave me a big hug. She was the nurse who'd screamed, "Give her some of the goddam hair!"

"Thank you for speaking up for me," I said.

She kept telling me how shocked she was, and for a few moments, I didn't understand. Then I did: Elizabeth's survival had shocked her—and though I felt momentarily that Elizabeth had survived all danger, I soon found out from the next visitor just how wrong I was.

CHAPTER 6

BACK TO THE WOODS

A nurse named Ally carried a big, white binder into Elizabeth's room. It contained, according to Ally, all the information I would need to help me understand what to expect in the coming days and weeks. As Ally guided me through the binder, the truth that Elizabeth was not yet out of the woods—not even close—began to sink in. My heart pounded in my throat, and tears gathered at the corners of my eyes.

"Just take it hour by hour," Ally told me, just as the TRU nurse had.

I learned about the two critical periods in the early recovery for a person with a brain injury. The initial critical period when injuries may be so bad that they cause death, even with the best care, occurs the first day or two after the injury. Those who survive this period face another critical period a few days later, lasting for approximately two more weeks during which time the brain may swell and complications occur at any time. Elizabeth had now entered into this second period.

I sat in the ICU, trying to find some part of my daughter's body that I could hold onto that didn't have a bandage on it or tube running into it. Our bleak reality and the uncertainty of my daughter's future expanded and filled my vision. Even if she lived, her education and her dreams felt gone. Would she ever be able to leave home and become an adult?

I felt enormous guilt for all the arguments we'd ever had. How I wished she could hear me say how much I loved her and how sorry I was for all the hostility! How had we even gotten here, a mother and daughter, fighting and hurting?

As an infant, Elizabeth had a big pudgy face with big, dark-brown eyes. Her hair stayed white-blonde until she was four years old, then turned golden. She loved the outdoors so much that you could call her a tomboy. From her adventures outside, many a frog, cricket, and gnarly spider entered our home with her help. With great excitement, she would show me what she'd found and ask if she could keep it. She filled jars with lightning bugs each summer night and placed them by her bedside to watch them glow. In the morning, after Elizabeth had punched holes in the jar's top so the bugs could breath, the bedroom would be filled with the rogue insects, trying to find their way back outside.

Because of their age difference, Elizabeth and Logan never really played together, but they shared a definite connection that held over the years. We had our ups and downs—raising a teenager and toddler at the same time was hard. To help out Frank, a self-employed contractor, I worked at a local bank.

We lived in Centreville then, a suburban town on the Eastern Shore of Maryland, in my dream home. Frank and I had wanted a house we could flip, but when we laid eyes on a neglected 19th-century house in 1996, we both saw its potential. The house was originally two buildings that had been pieced together; in the attic, you could see where the two roof tops met. We made an offer within days.

We moved in after 18 months of restoration when Elizabeth was three-and-a-half. It felt immediately like home. Elizabeth's large bedroom held lots of sunlight and stuffed animals; dusty pink walls framed windows with white curtains that touched the floor. Elizabeth's furniture consisted mostly of hand-me-downs from her brother along with her great-grandmother's white wicker rocking chair.

One night, while I lay on Elizabeth's bed, reading a book to her, she pointed upward and blurted, "Look, Mommy, there is someone watching us from the ceiling." I laughed and patted her hair, and then continued to read, but she pointed again and said, "Oh, they moved to Mama's chair."

I stopped reading, tried to stay calm, and asked her what she meant.

"A lady watches me at night, and she is here again."

I grabbed Elizabeth, ran out of her room, and sought out Frank.

"She watches too much Scooby Doo," he said and laughed.

As the days passed, I started to think that maybe he was right—I had made a big deal out of nothing. Then, a couple of weeks later, in the middle of the night when everyone was asleep, the sound of footsteps woke me—

three creaking sounds like someone was walking up the stairs. I lay in bed thinking I might be dreaming, but then I heard the sound again.

I woke Frank. He listened and agreed that he heard creaking sounds, too. He jumped out of bed and grabbed the baseball bat we kept by our bedside for protection. As he opened the door, he listened for the sound again. This time, we heard nothing. He started down the stairs, turning on every light switch as he stepped. Within five minutes, the house was lit up like a Christmas tree. I stood at the top of the stairs until I finally heard him say, "There is no one here."

From that moment on, we believed our house haunted. In the coming months, Elizabeth mentioned this lady many times. Even Logan's room emanated a lot of strange sounds heard only at night. Thankfully, he slept through the night, and the noises never affected him in any way.

Eventually, I decided I would talk to these "ghosts." I know it sounds ridiculous, but I felt I needed to do it in order to stay in the house. So, I went into Elizabeth's bedroom with a box of matches, thinking I would talk to the lady ghost of the house, you know, woman to woman.

I stood in the middle of her room, took out a match, and said in a firm voice, "Whoever you are, leave us alone, and don't hurt my kids. If you do, I will burn this house down. I promise you I will burn it down to the ground."

"We can share the house; there is plenty of room," I added. "Just leave us alone." From that day on, the house went silent.

Life seemed to be moving along just fine until we decided to move to a small, abandoned church building—a "fixer upper" Frank called it—on Tilghman Island, three square miles of land on the Chesapeake Bay. Before moving to Centreville, we had lived in a house close to the water, and ever since Frank had missed the convenience of walking down the road to get to his boat to go fishing and crabbing. The abandoned church building also had water access right down the road; that is why we purchased it. It was to be our weekend getaway until the kids moved out, and then it would become our retirement home.

Frank had started to restore the house, and I knew with his exceptional talents as a carpenter, the old church would become a lovely home for us. That happened sooner than planned, however. Logan enrolled in a community college in Annapolis and moved in with his mother who lived near this college. At that point, Frank pleaded for us to move, too. He really missed the water. Eager for him to be happy, I ultimately relented though moving so far away from our community concerned me. We put the Centreville house on the market.

Elizabeth and I went from the convenience of living in a town with shops, grocery stores, and the local library just a few blocks away to needing to drive 25 minutes for a gallon of milk. Frank spent most of his time working on the church, and on his days off, he just wanted to go fishing or rest. So, Elizabeth and I had only each other for company. We did everything together: shopping, riding bikes, and going to the beach at the end of our road for picnics.

Once Elizabeth started her new elementary school, a small school for the children on the island, she quickly became friends with the other students. She had no more than 20 classmates in her second-grade class. She seemed to be happy and adjusted just fine. Unfortunately, Frank and I had a less happy experience.

Once we moved to Tilghman Island, the cracks in our marriage began to show. Restoring the church took a lot more time and money than we had anticipated. I still worked for the same bank, though at a new branch, but I didn't make much. Tight money put an extra strain on our marriage. Frank seemed happy, but I missed the big, beautiful home we'd left behind in Centreville and grew resentful that I had given it up to live in the middle of nowhere. A magnificent place of water and sunsets in the summer, in the winter Tilghman Island gets cold, especially when the wind kicks up. When the tourists leave, the island feels deserted.

As the months passed, Frank and I fought every day. We began to realize that we'd had issues before the move to Tilghman Island but had simply been ignoring them. Considering it only a matter of time before one of us left the marriage, I made the decision to go.

Our separation devastated Elizabeth, then nine. Logan, already a grown man, worried more about his little sister, Elizabeth, who hoped we'd reunite. The separation, ugly at first, turned into a mutual decision by the time we divorced. Frank and I shared custody of Elizabeth, and she spent every other weekend with her dad, as well as a night or two during the week. She seemed to be handling the situation with resilience—until her teenage years.

Once Elizabeth turned 13, the closeness we had shared dissipated. I had remarried, and my second husband (Jim) and I lived in Easton with Elizabeth. The arguments and battles between Elizabeth and me subsumed our lives. At first, only typical teenage daughter complaints dominated: she felt I wanted to control her and raged that I wouldn't let her hang out with older kids or wear makeup. However, time revealed what fueled her anger: fury for leaving her father. She would scream at me that she hated me and would never forgive me for what I did to her father. She would also say how much she hated her new stepfather and how he would never replace her father. I do not regret getting a divorce, but I will always have misgivings about breaking up the family.

In the years that followed, my relationship with Elizabeth remained strained. We loved each other, but the bond I longed to have with her simply did not materialize. We learned to walk away from each other when our arguments got too heated, swallow hurtful words before expressing them, and cover over our feelings. She made little effort to get to know Jim. At best, she tolerated him. Jim tried his hardest to get Elizabeth to warm up to him through generosity with money and displayed great patience with her despite her icy attitude.

While Elizabeth's personality could be ugly at times, she had grown up to be stunningly beautiful, popular in high school, and the object of many boys' attention. She went to parties and high school sports games with her friends, got great grades, and was well known throughout her school as one of the "cool" kids.

In 10th grade, Elizabeth expressed interest in becoming a model. We signed her up at a modeling school in Wilmington, Delaware and every other Saturday for a year and a half, she and I made the two-hour drive so she could attend classes. The modeling school excited Elizabeth, and the drives gave us time to talk about her future and lay a better foundation. She would graduate from modeling school, finish high school, and then pursue her dream of becoming a model while taking community college courses.

Some of those dreams did come true. She finished modeling school. She experienced the normal teenage life: high school (an honor student), boyfriends, driver's license. Lying ahead: enrollment in community college and a modeling career.

~~~~~~~~~~~~~~~~

By Tuesday, three days after the accident, Elizabeth's condition had improved, if only slightly. The doctors told us that she was doing surprisingly well for a person who had suffered such severe injuries, but she remained in critical condition and on strong medications that prevented her from moving. Not moving also helped control her breathing (she was still on a ventilator), blood pressure, and other vital signs. She could, however, follow some commands. The nurses would ask her in a firm loud voice to move a finger, her toes, or squeeze a hand. If she could follow through on a command, this meant that the brain still functioned. That Elizabeth had followed a few commands gave hope.

I sat next to Elizabeth and told her how much I loved her and how proud I was of her for being so strong and brave. I sat in silence for a moment and heard the sounds of the machines keeping my daughter alive. Colored lines moved diagonally across screens. I heard the sound of a helicopter just outside our room then and went to the window. A medevac helicopter headed toward the hospital roof. As I lost sight of it, I put my hands together and prayed for the patient it carried—and the patient's family.

CHAPTER 7

STARTING A JOURNAL

Flipping through the big white binder on our fourth day in the hospital, I found a piece of paper with text on only one side. I sat by Elizabeth's bed, watching machines keep her broken body alive. Then, I flipped the paper over and started writing.

I do not particularly like to write. I've always been self-conscious about my poor grammar so I'd never kept a diary or journal of any type; even writing a simple thank-you note made me nervous. In that moment, though, I felt a strong urge to write down on paper everything stirring inside. I wanted to remember the details of what we were going through.

I filled that whole page and then wrote several more pages. The next day, I went to the hospital gift shop and purchased a small journal. As I wrote, I felt some of the overwhelming stress subside. I wrote more.

Soon, I decided to share some of my journal entries on a website called Caring Bridge the hospital had helped me set up for friends and family to access updates about Elizabeth. I wanted to give our community a firsthand account of our struggle and to help other young people like Elizabeth realize they were not invincible. Elizabeth had been careless when she drove that day, it was now clear, and I wanted other people her age to learn from her mistake. I would end each journal post with "Drive safely, and please pay attention behind the wheel" and sign each post as "Liz's mom"—how Elizabeth's friends would have thought of me.

The first journal post I shared was a note of gratitude. I thanked the responders to Elizabeth's car accident scene—the St. Michaels Volunteer

Fire Department, the paramedics, the Maryland State Police, the M.S.P. Medevac Unit, and everyone else. Their swift response enabled Elizabeth to receive the lifesaving treatment she needed.

I also thanked a gentleman named Robert Horton. I learned about him through a message his wife had sent to our family on a Facebook page set up by Elizabeth's friends. A man in his 40s with two teenage children, Robert was a construction worker who was working in the area near where the accident occurred. He and a co-worker heard a loud crash, stopped working to check it out, and then ran to the scene to help. The two men tried to open the driver's-side door on Elizabeth's car, but they couldn't. So, Robert opened her passenger door. He cut her seat belt with a buck knife so she could breathe. Then, he talked to her, telling her that help was on the way. Finally, he prayed for her.

I continued posting my journal entries on the Caring Bridge site about Elizabeth's serious condition and how she was not in the clear yet but that we were remaining strong and optimistic. We received the bad news that she had lost total sight in her left eye, but thankfully she could see out of her right one although the prognosis for her long-term vision in that eye was still unclear.

We thanked everyone for their prayers and hoped that the prayers would continue.

Elizabeth was off some of the sedating medications and now able to respond to more commands. She even got feisty with the nurses as they did certain procedures on her—a good sign, according to the nurses and doctors. By a week after her accident, the ventilator that helped Elizabeth breathe only provided her with supplemental oxygen. She now followed my commands. Feeling my daughter moving her hand in mine moved me to tears. It brought back memories of when she was a baby, reaching for her Mommy's hand for the first time and holding it for comfort and love.

Elizabeth never seemed to lie still. She constantly tried to pull out the tubes that kept her alive—so much so that the nurses had to put mittens on her hands. I could tell Elizabeth hated this because she was always trying to pull those off, too--unsuccessfully.

With tubes running down her throat, Elizabeth could not talk. Moreover, because of her traumatic brain injury, she might have to relearn *how* to talk, the doctors told us—she might be able to say some words, but they weren't sure how many. I talked to Elizabeth when I was next to her. I wanted her to know that I was with her and loved her. She was responding to my commands so I was hopeful that she recognized my voice.

When it came time for the nurses to perform procedures, I would get a cup of coffee and try to eat something. Unfortunately, I started smoking again. I had quit five years earlier and never thought I would start up again. I would also write in my journal about the day before, what progress Elizabeth had made, and how I felt. I wrote about the fears and demons that plagued me the most at night.

I really hated nights. One night I thought I had lost something precious of Elizabeth's: a necklace that Elizabeth had been wearing when she was admitted to the hospital.

I wrote about it in my journal, one of the first personal journal entries that I shared with everyone:

Dear Journal,

Earlier this evening in the hotel room, I was frantically looking for the necklace that was in the package I picked up from the hospital's bottom floor. Inside of it were all of Elizabeth's personal belongings that she was wearing when she was admitted to the hospital, including her high school class ring, earrings, and a necklace that I had given to her on her 13th birthday. The necklace was in the shape of two hearts intertwined together, which to me symbolized two sisters, one here on earth and the other in heaven. They may be separated, but their hearts and souls are forever together. When I gave it to Elizabeth, I told her the meaning behind the two hearts, and she just loved it. She put the necklace on and never took it off. She wore it every day from that birthday on.

Now, I couldn't find it. I don't know where I put it. I started to lose my composure. I began opening drawers and throwing clothes everywhere. I looked inside my purse several times but still could not find it.

Jim told me to not worry, that we would find it. My mom asked me if I had looked in my purse, and I screamed at her, "Of course, I did!"

She told me to look one more time, "Dump everything out of your purse onto the bed."   As I did this, the necklace fell out of the purse and onto the bed. I remember grabbing the necklace. hugging my mom, and saying that I was sorry. I took the necklace into the bathroom, shut the door behind me, and held the necklace in my hand. I thanked God that I had found it.

That is when I noticed my daughter's blood on the necklace. I immediately started to wash the blood off. As I was watching the water stream down on the necklace, I saw bloody water gushing down the drain. I felt pain and extreme sadness. I took a towel and dried off the necklace and remember feeling totally broken. I thought to myself: this is going to be another long night for me.

Drive safely, and please pay attention behind the wheel.
Liz's Mom

Part Two

RECOVERY

"An injury is not just a process of recovery; it is a process of discovery."
Conor McGregor

Betty Shaw

CHAPTER 8

A GRANOLA BAR

The damage to Elizabeth's face, according to the plastic surgeons at Shock Trauma, was "among the worst" they had ever seen. She had bone fragments scattered under her skin and major bone displacement of her left eye socket and left cheekbone. Everyone on her plastics team agreed that if they were not treated immediately, her facial injuries could kill her. The team scheduled her first facial reconstructive surgery for April 15, just eight days after her accident.

I woke early on the day of Elizabeth's first reconstructive surgery after tossing and turning all night long without any restful sleep. I made coffee, poured it into a thermos, and put it, along with snacks, my journal, and my Bible into the backpack-like-purse that had become my hospital bag. I'd lost count of how many times I had pulled out the Bible, held Dad's and Elizabeth's hair in my hands, and prayed for a miracle.

As I now did every morning, I sat outside in front of the hotel near some small tables and chairs for guests. I picked the table farthest from the other tables so I could avoid the need to make small talk. I wrote in my journal and lit up a cigarette. I knew I needed to stop smoking, but it had become an escape for me, a stress-release, like doing something you knew you're not supposed to do but you don't care. If not smoking, then drinking—and I knew I couldn't function if drunk all the time. So, I told myself that after Elizabeth returned home and all the current trauma had passed, I would never light up again.

My cell phone rang. Dr. Amir Dorafshar, a plastic surgeon at Shock Trauma, who would perform Elizabeth's reconstructive surgery, wanted to touch base. One of the world's most renowned plastic surgeons, just the March before Elizabeth's car accident, as part of a plastics surgical team, he had helped to perform the most extensive successful face transplant to date. Dr. Dorafshar went over what he would accomplish for Elizabeth during her surgery. He told me many procedures would be performed, taking up to eight hours. He then prepared me for everything that could potentially go wrong—and I started to cry.

At that point, Dr. Dorafshar stopped talking about what could go wrong and assured me in a voice filled with confidence and sincerity that he would treat my daughter as if she were his own. Although I had not met Dr. Dorafshar in person, I instinctively felt that I was placing Elizabeth in the right hands.

~~~~~~~~~~~~~~~

Following that conversation, Jim and I walked to the hospital to begin our long day of waiting out Elizabeth's surgery. Along the way, a homeless man approached me and held out his hand for money. Many times, on my daily walks to the hospital, homeless people would ask me for change or a cigarette, and I'd given a little money and a lot of my cigs to them. As this man spoke to me, though, my heart was closed to him. I felt no true compassion. He chose to live this kind of life, and if he really wanted to, he could just stop. I hurried on toward my daughter and never gave the man another thought.

Elizabeth's surgery didn't get started until 8:45 a.m., and by the 8-hour mark, at 4:45 in the afternoon, the surgery was still not over. Elizabeth would never look the way she had before the car accident, and I knew it would take years of surgeries even to get close to regaining her appearance. It scared me to think about how hard it was going to be for this once very attractive young girl to be blind in one eye and have a disfigured face. I just hoped that one day she would be able look in the mirror and be happy with her reflection.

Nine hours went by. Ten. Soon, it would be 11.

At last, Dr. Dorafshar came out to the waiting area. "She is stable and resting," he said. "I pieced her face back together as best as I could, and I think you will be happy with the results. I was actually able to perform several procedures in this one interval," he continued. "That's why it took so much longer than we expected."

I couldn't believe it. I hugged him, and he hugged me back. I felt the goodness in his soul—and so did all the rest of the family. All of us, who had been waiting out Elizabeth's surgery, surrounded Dr. Dorafshar. Overjoyed, amazed, and grateful, every single one hugged and thanked him—and felt warmed by his smile. With Elizabeth's reconstructive surgery behind her and the surgeons and other doctors happy with the results, I wanted to do something to thank everyone one of them—Drs. Dorafshar and Sutcliffe, the surgeons (including, especially, Dr. Aaron), the interns, the nurses, and every single other person who had made a difference in Elizabeth's life—but the nurse on duty at the station told me the hospital did not allow anyone on staff to accept gifts.

"How about food?" I asked. "I bake a mean brownie."

"Stop right there," she said. "We love food."

I went straight to the Caring Bridge site and asked our community for help. After all, people had been asking constantly if there was anything they could do for us. I also asked them to put a thank you note with their baked goods for the doctors and nurses who were taking care of Elizabeth.

A few days later, my mom met me at the hotel. I just cried when I saw her car filled to capacity with baked goods: cookies, brownies, even Danishes—so many items it took me about two hours to hand-deliver the pastries to each of the six floors of the Shock Trauma Unit. Later, when I peeked out from Elizabeth's room, I saw that some of the nurses reading the cards had tears in their eyes.

~~~~~~~~~~~~~~

Elizabeth turned 18 in the ICU on April 22nd. She still could not speak but was improving every day. The tube draining the fluid from her brain had been removed, and she had been taken off the ventilator. Her scalp started to grow new hair. Her face appeared less swollen, and she seemed to be in less pain. She still tried to remove her tubes and started to scratch the stitches on her head—179 in all—so much so that the nurses had to put white gloves over her hands or even restrain her arms. They nicknamed her "Squirmy."

I sat next to her and read aloud the many birthday cards family and friends had sent, more than 100. She did not understand what I was reading. She would just grab a card and hand it back to me, but I think she looked at the pictures.

I had never dreamed that we would be celebrating her 18th birthday—or any birthday—in an ICU. I still wanted to know what had she been doing behind the wheel that caused her to sustain so much damage to her body. Undoubtedly, she was not paying attention, but a lot of people don't pay attention when they are driving. Many people drive drunk and yet make it safely home. Why are they not punished each time? Why, God, did you choose Elizabeth to punish? Why did you pick a young, loving, and good girl and not some drug addict or serial killer to go through this kind of hell?

I was still feeling sorry for myself later that afternoon while waiting in the hospital lobby for an elevator to go back upstairs to Elizabeth's room when I happened to overhear an older gentleman, about 70, asking how to get to Shock Trauma's ICU on the fourth floor.

"I'm on my way there," I said. "You can follow me."

"Wonderful," he said. "Thanks so much."

"Who are you here to see?" I asked, after pressing the button.

"My great-niece," he replied. "She was in a very bad car accident. It does not look good." He looked at the ground and rubbed his hands along the sides of his pants.

"I'm so sorry," I said. "My daughter was in a bad car accident, too. Her outcome looked really bleak when we first got here, but amazing things happen in this hospital. She is doing well. Hang in there. I will pray for a miracle for your great-niece."

"Thank you," he said and accepted the hug I was offering.

When the elevator doors opened, we went our separate ways.

Later, as I was walking around Elizabeth's floor, I noticed that two doors down from Elizabeth was a 19-year-old girl. Nurses and doctors bustled in and out of her room. I wondered what had happened to her.

~~~~~~~~~~~~~~~

A few days later, I was hanging out in the waiting room and writing in my journal while Elizabeth was having a physical therapy session. These sessions were hard to watch—the nurses moved parts of her body around to help with blood flow, but I could tell it was very painful for her.

"Do you know if there is any place in the hospital that sells soup?" a woman asked me. She had been sitting in the waiting room with me, but I'd hardly noticed her.

Right away I knew that whomever she was there to see was not in good shape. When Elizabeth first got to Shock Trauma, the only thing I could eat was soup. It was easy and quick to swallow; it was something to survive on.

I told the woman where to go and asked her if she needed any help in getting there, but she declined my assistance. Later, when we saw each other inside the ICU unit, we exchanged smiles.

The next day when I was visiting Elizabeth, there was a light knock on Elizabeth's open door.

"May I come in?" asked this same woman.

"Yes, of course, please come in," I said. She introduced herself as Mary and thanked me for helping her uncle a few days earlier—the man from the elevator.

"Of course," I said. "How is she? Whoever you're here for, I mean."

"My daughter," she said. "She was in a car accident, and it looks very bad for her."

I found another chair and put it next to mine. "Sit down, please," I said.

I grabbed her hand and told her about what had happened to Elizabeth and how grim things had looked for her. I also told her that her daughter was in a great hospital, receiving premier care. I shared with her how the doctors and nurses miraculously saved Elizabeth's life. I told her to hang in there and not to give up hope. She smiled weakly.

Mary told me how her daughter had been a passenger in a car driven by a friend who ran a red light. Another car hit his car, with Mary's daughter in its front passenger seat—the area that took most of the impact. The driver of the car walked away from the accident without a scratch, as did a passenger in the back seat. Mary's daughter's spine was crushed beyond repair, and she would be paralyzed from the neck down for the rest of her life.

There was nothing I could say. I just grabbed her and held on to her as she cried.

A few nights later when I was leaving the hospital, I walked past the room of Mary's daughter. I usually didn't look into the rooms of other patients because I thought that would be rude, but on this night, I did look for just a second.

Mary's daughter was alone, strapped to a bed that was almost vertical like she was in a standing position. I heard the sounds of all the machines connected to this girl's body just like they had been connected to Elizabeth when she was first admitted to the ICU. I looked into Mary's daughter's eyes and gave her a quick smile. Then, I continued walking.

After that, I stopped feeling as sorry for myself. I no longer felt angry at the world. That night, I prayed for a miracle to happen for Mary's daughter.

~~~~~~~~~~~~~~

I kept seeing the homeless people on my walks to the hospital. Sometimes when I was outside smoking in the park in front of the hospital, I would even have a conversation with one or two of them. Eventually, I became comfortable enough around them to ask some questions. How did you become homeless? Do you have family that is worried about you? Where do you sleep at night? Many of them were too drunk or too high to answer, but some did.

One young woman, perhaps 30, told me that she had been in a car accident and had broken her back, then became addicted to painkillers. She started to steal from her family and friends to get her next high, and soon her parents kicked her out of their home. Her friends helped her out for a while, but they kicked her out as well. Then, she went on the streets. I could tell that she had been very attractive at one time, but now she was wearing torn, dirty clothes and hadn't bathed in months. I wanted to give her money, but I stopped myself. I knew she would use it for drugs. We said our goodbyes, and I returned to the hospital.

Sitting next to Elizabeth, I made a note to myself to buy and always carry granola bars with me so that I would have something to give to any homeless person who asked for money for food.

I went through many packages of granola bars after that. Whenever a homeless person would ask me for money to buy food, I would hold out a granola bar instead. Most of the time this worked; the person would thank me and walk away. I did have the occasional granola bar thrown back in my face, but I didn't get mad. I began to feel sympathy for them. Many came from abusive family situations. Others had no family at all. Drugs and alcohol were the only way they knew how to cope with their physical pain—and then their addiction became their new inner pain, something that not only controlled their lives but also destroyed them.

CHAPTER 9

STORMS

Three and a half weeks after the accident, Elizabeth was finally moved out of the ICU to the sixth floor of Shock Trauma where she would await transfer to Kennedy Krieger Institute (KKI for short), the brain rehabilitation center of Johns Hopkins. Though Elizabeth had turned 18 and the institute was for children 17 and younger, we thought she could relate better with patients closer to her age. Plus, it sits on the east side of Baltimore, just a few minutes from Shock Trauma.

Elizabeth had been having what the doctors called "brain storms." When one hit, her whole body would stiffen so rigidly that we could not bend it, and her jaw would clamp shut. The nurses and I would try to massage her muscles to relax them and reassure her that the storm would be over soon. Doctors told us that this was a normal part of Elizabeth's brain recovery process, proof that her undamaged brain tissue cells were gradually learning how to perform some of the functions of the destroyed cells. I could see by the look on her face, though, that these "storms" caused her extreme pain—and the pain medication ordered for them did not control the pain enough.

After each brain storm, I noticed Elizabeth becoming more aware of her surroundings. At times, she looked scared to death, like she had no idea how she'd ended up in a hospital bed. I would reassure her that she was fine, that she had been in a car accident and was being well cared for at the hospital. She would look at me and seem to understand, but an hour later, that same scared look would reappear on her face. It had gotten to the point where I would have to tell her the story of her accident every hour. Her battered brain could not hold onto the message.

I brought Elizabeth some blank writing paper and encouraged her to try to write or draw. At first, she managed only a scribble, but with each passing day, she improved. I asked her simple questions and showed her how to write the answers down on the paper. When she tried to write words, though, I could not read her handwriting—or doodling—and this frustrated her.

Late in the evening on what I thought would be Elizabeth's last day in the hospital before transferring to KKI, I was once again telling her where she was and how she got there when I noticed her getting very agitated. While I was still speaking, she grabbed a piece of writing paper and a pen. She scrawled something on the paper, then handed it to me.

I looked at the paper. She had written words. They read:

"Get it."

My heart surged with joy. My daughter was still in there—badly damaged, but still there and letting me know that she understood what I had been telling her about being in the hospital and about how she got there. Finally, validation! I still have that piece of paper! I always will!

~~~~~~~~~~~~~~~

After four days on the sixth floor, Elizabeth still had not been transferred. The supervisor told me lack of a patient opening caused the delay, but I grew impatient and frustrated. I felt Elizabeth was not receiving the care she had gotten in the ICU so I stayed by her side around the clock. I pulled up a chair next to her bed and slept there though I never truly slept—whenever the nurses came in to check on Elizabeth, it woke me. Elizabeth became restless whenever her diaper was full and needed to be changed. I would notify a nurse immediately, but it took too long for one to show up and help. To speed things up, I started to change my daughter's diapers myself. With each diaper change, I found myself getting more and more depressed. Memories of changing her diaper as an infant flooded through my mind. I never imagined that I would be doing it again when she was 18 years old.

I grew nasty toward the nurses. I even complained to the nurses' supervisor about how I felt they were not attending to Elizabeth the way they should have been. The supervisor listened patiently to my complaints, then reminded me that my daughter was not the only patient requiring nursing care.

As a result, however, the hospital did assign a nurse's aide to be at Elizabeth's side at all times. I was very grateful and apologized to the nurses for my behavior. Now that someone would be with Elizabeth, I decided to return to the hotel to get much-needed sleep. I gave Elizabeth a hug goodbye and told her I would be back later. She put her arms around me and wouldn't let go. She was trying to say something, but I couldn't understand her. She started to get upset. I looked at the nurse's aide.

"Leave, and get some rest," she said. She assured me she would take good care of Elizabeth and reminded me that I needed to take care of myself as well. I pulled Elizabeth's arms off of me and left without looking back. When I made it outside, my face was wet with tears.

When I got to the hotel room, I was still crying so loudly that I put a bathroom towel over my face to muffle the sound. Then, I collapsed on the bed.

The next thing I remember is waking up three hours later to the sound of my cell phone ringing. The supervisor in charge of Elizabeth's transfer informed me that Elizabeth would be going to the brain rehab center within the hour.

When I called Jim with the good news, he joked, "The transfer was probably expedited not because of her but because they wanted to get rid of her mother!" Probably spot on!

CHAPTER 10
THE TEXT

After attending Elizabeth's high school graduation on her behalf as well as a fundraiser our community held for St. Michaels Fire Department in Elizabeth's honor, I prepared to return to Baltimore, when I decided to stop by the Maryland State Police Barracks, located just a few miles from our home. I wanted to let the officer who came to our door on that terrible day know that Elizabeth was at a brain rehab center recovering from her injuries and to apologize for screaming at him when it must have been so difficult to deliver such bad news.

When I arrived at the barracks, the officer wasn't there. Seeing my disappointment, the woman at the desk told me that Officer Gates, the investigating officer for Elizabeth's accident, was in the building. I asked if I could see him. I thought maybe he could shed some light on what had caused the accident.

Officer Gates told me that he had been the first to arrive at the scene. The car lay wrecked and smoking, and he knew right away that the young girl in the car had a very slim chance of survival. Officer Gates had approached the car and noticed Robert Horton, the man who had been doing construction work nearby, in the car, rescuing Elizabeth. Asked if Elizabeth was alive, Mr. Horton replied she was breathing—but barely.

Officer Gates wondered whether it was even worth calling for a medevac, but the weather that day was sunny and the skies exceptionally clear. So, he took a chance and called. He said that if it had been a rainy or overcast day he would not have done so—weather systems make the medevac's job harder and slower. My daughter's life would not have been saved had it not been for the good weather and this officer who made that call. My knees started to buckle.

"Are you alright?" asked Officer Gates. He led me toward a meeting room where we could continue our conversation.

"Thank you so much," I told him, once we were seated. "I'm so thankful you made that choice, and I'm so grateful to the officer who came to our door to tell me about Elizabeth's accident."

Officer Gates just nodded. Then, he told me that he had found Elizabeth's purse and in it her driver's license and had recognized her name. His niece and Elizabeth were high school friends. He said he feared that Elizabeth would not survive so he had sent the other officer to tell us of the accident in person.

Again, I thanked him. I told him how Elizabeth was now being cared for in a brain rehab facility and how her progress had been encouraging the doctors. She had a long road of recovery ahead of her, but her future looked promising. Officer Gates told me he had been reading about her in the local paper and was amazed she was doing so well.

In the silence that followed, I worked up my courage. "What was she doing when the accident happened?" I asked. "Do you know?"

"Yes," he said. "She was texting and driving. We found her cell phone on the front passenger floorboard. When the impact occurred, her head was facing downward, and there were no brake marks on the road." He paused, then added, "The cell phone your daughter had in her hand caused her accident. We didn't subpoena her phone because I was 99% certain she was texting and driving. I never bothered to follow through on that issue because I didn't think she would live."

"I can't believe she would do that," I said. "I warned her about the danger of using her cell phone behind the wheel. She promised me she never did."

"I'm sorry," he said. "Our investigation revealed otherwise."

~~~~~~~~~~~~~~

I drove straight back to our house and found Elizabeth's cell phone. At home the day before, I noticed that her pink overnight bag had been returned, and someone—probably Jim—had placed it on her bed.

I opened the bag. Inside lay her school books, laptop, clothes, and cell phone. The cell phone needed to be charged. As I waited, I became madder and madder at the person that she was texting. I wanted to know what kind of conversation was so important that Elizabeth had nearly died for it. I was going to make that person feel very deep guilt and remorse for what they had done not only to Elizabeth but also to her family.

Once the cell phone turned on, I thumbed through her text messages, looking for the last opened or sent message. It didn't take long. It was an incoming message at 10:52 a.m., and it read: "OK." Then, to my horror, I realized I had sent that message. I was responding to her text sent moments earlier, telling me that she wouldn't be able to make it back home before work that morning.

"Oh, my God!" I gasped. "She was reading *my* text message!" *I* was my daughter's distraction. *I* was the one who had destroyed her life.

I checked her phone again, frantically hoping to find another subsequently opened or sent message from someone else. As I was thumbing through, I prayed to God *please do not let it be me*. But it was. There was no way to make it not be true. Disbelief, then shame engulfed me. There I was, writing to Elizabeth's young friends, telling them to pay attention behind the wheel and drive safely when it was an adult, her mother, who had caused the accident.

How could a mother send an inexperienced 17-year-old driver a text message? Even though Elizabeth had told me she never used her phone when she was driving, as a parent, I should not have given her any temptation.

Back in Baltimore, I didn't tell Jim what I had learned. I didn't have the courage or the energy to deal with his reaction on learning the awful truth. Each morning after that, I awoke washed in guilt and shame. Those feelings followed me throughout the day from when I woke up until I put my head down to sleep. I decided I would keep this shameful secret to myself forever, that I would take it to the grave.

CHAPTER 11
MAJOR COMPLICATION

At KKI, Elizabeth had two sitters assigned to watch over her morning, afternoon, and night to make sure she was safe, comfortable and that she didn't pull out her tubes. Despite her improvement, she still had a feeding tube, a trachea, and an IV for fluids and antibiotics to prevent infections.

The plan we'd settled on with her KKI medical team meant that Elizabeth would go through intense brain rehabilitation and physical rehabilitation, with the goal to be released from the KKI within six weeks, after which she would receive outpatient rehabilitation. Only *six weeks,* and she could be home—incredible! The doctors assured us that it was an achievable goal and that KKI could make it happen.

As the nurses helped Elizabeth settle into her new surroundings, I filled her room with cards and posters from well-wishers so Elizabeth could see from her bed that she was loved. I brought her a gift her high school classmates made for her: a box shaped like a graduation cap filled with letters from each of her fellow graduating students. A week earlier, I had watched Elizabeth's friends and fellow classmates cross the stage and receive their diplomas with pride and joy on their faces and felt the sting of sadness that Elizabeth was missing this pivotal moment.

Elizabeth was doing well in all her therapy classes, but she still had difficulty accepting solid foods into her mouth. With extreme patience, the nurses and I tried to reteach her how to eat, but she resisted. During her down time, she loved to ride in her wheelchair and be pushed around the hallways so she could wave to everyone she saw. She still could not speak because of the trach tube, but that didn't stop her from trying to make friends.

~~~~~~~~~~~~~~

With Elizabeth in the capable hands of her sitters and the medical staff at KKI, we settled our bill at the hotel and took my sister-in-law up on her offer for us to stay at her home in Glen Burnie, on the outskirts of Baltimore, for the next six weeks.

When Elizabeth had been at KKI for a week, I arrived around 10:30 one morning after running errands and sat down in the room where she was having her therapy session. I watched her progress. After a few moments, I noticed something strange about the left side of her face and interrupted the therapist.

"Does it look a little swollen to you?" I asked.

The therapist looked at Elizabeth's face. "You know, you're right," she said.

She stopped the session and called a nurse. The nurse looked at Elizabeth and decided she needed to be seen by a doctor. Elizabeth was returned to her room, and we waited for an hour for the doctor to examine her, only to be told she needed to be seen back at Shock Trauma because they were more familiar with her case.

We waited more than six hours for the transfer. With every passing minute, Elizabeth's face became more and more swollen. By the time we made it back to Shock Trauma, at 6:00 p.m., I was seething with anger and frustration.

The ambulance pulled up to the emergency entrance of the hospital where a male nurse met us and transferred Elizabeth off the gurney and onto a hospital bed. He took Elizabeth back to the TRU (Trauma Resuscitation Unit) floor, where she had first arrived when flown into Shock Trauma.

"It's going to be chaotic," he said. "Not as bad as when she first arrived, but they will have to do many tests to determine her current condition."

I braced myself. As the elevator doors opened, memories of what we had gone through five weeks earlier flooded back. I saw the cubicle where we prayed and where Elizabeth's blood had covered the floor. I heard the beeps of the emergency machines and felt sick to my stomach.

The doctor didn't come to speak with us until the middle of the night. The hospital was quieter by then. Frank, Jim, and I sat next to each other in Elizabeth's cubicle, not leaving her side, waiting for her return the few times she was taken away for CT scans and other testing. Frank and Jim made small talk, but I sat there, holding Elizabeth's hand, focused intently on her, and watched her become less and less responsive—until the doctor appeared at 2:00 a.m.

"Elizabeth has developed an infection in the areas around her face and scalp that were damaged from the car accident," the doctor said. "The infection has not spread into the brain, and I don't feel there is a need for surgery at this time. We'll put her on a strong dose of antibiotics—three different kinds; the combination should reduce the spreading and clear the infection."

Elizabeth was readmitted into the hospital to be monitored for a day or so before being cleared to return to the KKI. Back we went to the sixth floor, the floor where I was so nasty to the nurses. After Elizabeth was admitted, Frank went home, and Jim and I went back to our hotel to get some sleep. I returned to the hospital alone the next day at 11:00 a.m. to be by Elizabeth's side, Jim having to go to work. Based on what the doctors had told us, I had expected to see some improvement in Elizabeth's condition. Conversely, I noticed a big decline in her demeanor. Worrisomely, she had become very lethargic. I found Bob, the nurse assigned to her, and expressed my concern. He agreed with me and told me that when he'd started his shift earlier that morning, Elizabeth was squirmy and agitated but as the morning passed had become still and non-responsive. Though she had stable vital signs, something just didn't seem right. Bob got on the phone right away.

A half-hour later, Dr. Dorafshar stood outside Elizabeth's room. We hadn't seen him since Elizabeth's marathon reconstructive surgery, and as he entered, relief swept over me. He went over to examine Elizabeth. I watched him for any signs of concern, but his face never changed. Not yet 40 years old, with glasses and curly black hair, he exuded great confidence. Then, he spoke, in the optimistic and reassuring voice that I had come to trust.

"Twenty percent of patients with severe brain injuries develop infections around the damaged areas," he said. "Unfortunately, Elizabeth is one of these patients."

Dr. Dorafshar started to say more, but right then, Dr. Aaron, Elizabeth's neurosurgeon, appeared outside the door and requested a meeting with Dr. Dorafshar. Within ten minutes, I sat talking with both surgeons and a half dozen other people in a conference room, including the chief doctor of the sixth floor, Dr. Bolander. Dr. Bolander started by saying that

Elizabeth was not responding to the antibiotics, which made him seriously concerned about her condition. He thought that Elizabeth should go into surgery and have the infected areas cleared out to help the antibiotics work better.

Dr. Aaron, seated across from me, spoke next. He wore a sweater vest over a short-sleeved shirt and spoke with a German accent. He recommended putting Elizabeth on stronger antibiotics and waiting to see if she responded. Dr. Bolander and Dr. Aaron went back and forth on what each one considered best for Elizabeth.

Then, Dr. Bolander asked Dr. Dorafshar for his opinion. Dr. Dorafshar sat next to me, a few chairs down from the other two doctors.

"I agree with Dr. Bolander," he said in a confident, calm, and respectful manner. He went on to explain how antibiotics do not respond well in the presence of excess pus in affected areas. He recommended surgery to clear all the affected areas and then putting Elizabeth on stronger antibiotics.

Dr. Aaron looked straight at me then and told me in a firm voice, "We could lose her." He felt that going back in could result in further complications, and he strongly opposed it. My shoulders slumped, but I maintained my cool. I knew that a decision had to be made and that I had to make it.

The room fell silent as everyone waited for my response. I turned and looked at Dr. Dorafshar. "Take her now," I said. "She doesn't look good to me." The confidence with which Dr. Dorafshar had given his opinion, coupled with what he had already done for my daughter by repairing her face in just one surgery, made me decide to go with my gut feeling of trust in this doctor.

As it turned out, no surgery rooms were available until 8:00 the following morning. Here we were talking about the seriousness of Elizabeth's condition, and now she could not get surgery right away. The doctors assured me her vital signs were stable so we had time. I felt gravely concerned that she would fade with each passing hour. Again, I feared I would lose her.

No one spoke as we left the meeting room. I knew my decision had disappointed Dr. Aaron. Dr. Dorafshar came up and gave me a hug and reassured me he would take good care of Elizabeth. Once again, I felt that whatever the outcome was, my decision to trust him had been the right one.

I went to that same small park in front of the hospital where I had already spent so much time. I wanted to have a good cry. In the park, I had occasionally seen rats running about during the day looking for food scraps, but I didn't care. The green grass and plants reminded me of home. I sat down on a bench, pulled out a cigarette, and lit it up.

As I sat there, once again feeling sorry for myself, a homeless woman with matted hair and a slightly harsh aroma sat down on the other end of the bench and asked me if I had a cigarette to spare. I gave her one.

When I handed it to her, she noticed that I was crying. She asked me what I was crying about, and I told her about Elizabeth and the meeting.

"Let's pray," she said.

Though leery about her motives, I felt desperate so I put my head down, and she began to pray for me. She spoke out loud, asking God to help my daughter and to make everything better for me. It was unbelievable. Here was a woman with everything to her name gathered next to her in two bags, no home to call her own, and no idea where she would get her next meal praying for Elizabeth and me.

As I listened, I felt horrible for the way I'd questioned her motives. Further, I was lucky to have had Elizabeth for 18 years, and so far, she was still with me. I had food on my table and a warm bed to rest my head each night. By the end of the prayer, I felt fortunate and blessed. Even at this time of hardship in my life, I was sure I experienced no hardship compared to what this poor woman was living through.

My cell phone rang. The lead nurse from the meeting told me that they were taking Elizabeth into surgery at that moment.

"How is that possible?" I asked.

"An opening came up," she said. "A patient chewed gum before his scheduled surgery so it had to be postponed."

I couldn't believe it! A miracle had just happened, and I felt sure it was because of the kind-hearted lost soul sitting next to me in the park. I hung up the phone, told the woman what had just happened, and gave her a big hug. I thanked her for her prayer and told her she would be in my prayers from then on. Before I left, I gave her all the cigarettes I had left.

Betty Shaw

CHAPTER 12

HOMECOMING

I made it back in time to give Elizabeth a quick kiss goodbye, and then she was taken away for surgery. I noticed both Dr. Dorafshar and Dr. Aaron following her as she was being wheeled to those now sadly familiar double doors. Bob told me that both doctors would be in surgery with Elizabeth. Dr. Dorafshar would perform the surgery, and Dr. Aaron would stand by in case he might be needed.

Wow, I just rejected Dr. Aaron's decision, yet he's still taking care of my daughter! That was the first time I realized while doctors have different opinions about best treatment, they will put aside any disappointment if their opinion does not prevail and do their best to ensure a patient's well-being.

With Elizabeth on the way to surgery, I called Jim and Frank. Both were on their way, and within 90 minutes, the three of us were in a waiting room, anticipating word of the result of the surgery.

My cell phone rang: Dr. Dorafshar. "The surgery went well," he said. "I removed all the infection, and she is now resting peacefully in recovery. You can see her soon."

"Thank you, Dr. Dorafshar. Please tell Dr. Aaron we thank him as well."

"He has already left the hospital," Dr. Dorafshar informed me. Unfortunately, we never got the chance to thank Dr. Aaron in person.

We returned to Elizabeth's side and noticed right away a more responsive, though still groggy, demeanor. In the following days, she became more alert—and squirmier. Her doctor decided she was well enough to be put into a cage-like tent so she could move around more freely yet remain safe. Every two hours or so, a nurse and I would take her out of the tent and help her walk around the hospital floor hallways. She loved this. She would wave to everyone just like she did when she was in her wheelchair at KKI.

On her last night in Shock Trauma before she was to return to KKI, a female nurse and I were walking Elizabeth around the hallways when a really cute male nurse walked past us. Elizabeth stopped in her tracks, watching him, then turned her body so she could keep looking at him with her one good eye. After he'd walked away, Elizabeth motioned for me and the female nurse to follow him. The nurse and I started to laugh.

"No can do," I told Elizabeth.

~~~~~~~~~~~~~~~

After finishing Elizabeth's walk, we put her back into her tent. Jim arrived to watch over Elizabeth while I got something to eat. I gave her a pad of paper and a pencil and told her to draw something for her stepdad. (Since she could not speak because of her trach tube, I continued to encourage her to write down what she wanted to say instead.) When I returned, my husband showed me what Elizabeth had written: "Where that guy?"

After some discussion, Jim told me that she was trying to say: "Where's that guy?" I took the note to the nurse's station and asked one of the female nurses for the name of the cute male nurse.

"We call him 'Nurse Cupcake,'" the nurse at the station told me. "Because he is so sweet to look at."

This was Elizabeth's last night on Shock Trauma's sixth floor. The next day, she returned to KKI by ambulance, with me in tow.

Once again settled into her KKI room, Elizabeth readied to restart her recovery. Increasingly attentive in her cognitive classes, she still struggled with her physical therapy classes. She had lost a lot of weight and strength. Moreover, like other brain-injury patients, she had trouble sleeping. Routinely unable to achieve REM sleep, she was often agitated and exhausted throughout the day. As well, she still had her feeding tube, which she hated. Her sitters often had to battle with her to get her to stop trying to pull it out; once again they encased her hands in mittens. Nonetheless, we were told that, all in all, she was doing well.

~~~~~~~~~~~~~~~

Next, Elizabeth started to play board games; her favorite game was UNO. She started remembering people and her surroundings. She started to read some of the many notes of encouragement and love sent to her through the Caring Bridge website. She understood what was being written to her and wanted to respond.

What's up? Soooo what's up with you all be awesome?!?! It's so FUNNY. I love you guys :)

She handed me this note one day and wanted me to post it. Even though it was hard to understand, I posted it exactly as it was. Everyone was excited to hear from her. Many people encouraged her to write even more.

I didn't allow mirrors in Elizabeth's room for fear of how she would react if she saw herself in the mirror, but that day had to come. It came when Elizabeth was able to use the bathroom once again. Her bathroom had a mirror, of course.

One morning after she used the toilet, instead of handing her a baby wipe to clean her hands, I guided her to the sink. Together we turned on the water. She played with the faucet for a while, and then I told her to look at the mirror.

She saw herself. She placed her hands on her head, moved them around, and felt the stubble of her hair. I told her it would grow back. Then, she leaned in closer and looked at her eyes. I waited for her to get upset, but she didn't say a word. Next, she turned her body around to look at her butt, did a little booty shake, and gave me a big smile. She turned away from the mirror and reached for the door.

I was shocked. The nurses reminded me, however, that cognitively Elizabeth still had a long way to go and that this was a typical reaction for many patients. It would take many more months before she became fully aware of what had happened to her.

We realized the difficulty of the months ahead almost immediately. As a result of the strong antibiotics that can cause yeast to grow out of control, Elizabeth developed thrush (a yeast infection of the mouth)—and from that, she lost more weight, grew weaker, and refused to eat through her mouth. She still had a feeding tube so she had a way to receive nutrition, but the lack of immediate diagnosis of thrush complicated the overall situation, causing Elizabeth to lose ground in her recovery. Once the KKI doctors had examined Elizabeth, found the thrush, and started treatment, Elizabeth began to put on weight and tried to communicate through moans and grunts.

With the KKI doctors noticing Elizabeth's attempts at communicating, using her hands and grunts, they decided the time had arrived to provide her with a speaking valve that fit over the protruding portion of the tube and allowed her, at last, to speak. Up until then, though, she had been fit with a trach tube following the tracheotomy right after her accident that allowed her to breathe and live, the trach tube was first connected to a ventilator. During that period of time, the trach tube and trachea would naturally become clogged from mucus that had to be suctioned out; the trach tube, too, needed to be periodically cleaned and regularly replaced with a new one. Although the doctors and nurses described these procedures as routine, they created some nervous moments for me, knowing that Elizabeth needed a clear airway at all times to breathe and stay alive. Although Elizabeth had been taken off the ventilator once she could breathe on her own, the trach tube remained; her dependency on it continued even as she was transferred to KKI Rehab.

Finally, the day came for her to be fitted with a speaking valve, a device enabling her to use her voice and therapy sessions to teach her how to use it. The therapist placed the device over the tracheal opening in Elizabeth's throat, then asked her to use her voice to recite the alphabet. At first, her voice sounded soft, like a whisper.

"Louder," the therapist said. Her ABCs were scratchy-sounding but when she heard her own voice for the first time, Elizabeth's face lit up. Sitting in a chair across the room, when I heard her voice for the first time, tears sprang to my eyes. I hadn't realized how much I missed hearing her voice.

Elizabeth continued to the end of the alphabet. Although she missed quite a few of the letters, no one in the room cared.

Elizabeth saw my tears and grabbed a tissue from a tissue box near her. She walked over, handed me the tissue, and asked me in her raspy voice, "Why are you crying, Mommy?"

Hearing her call me "Mommy" went straight to my soul.

Then, Elizabeth asked me if she had cancer like Pop-Pop? This shocked me. Was she in contact with my dad somehow? I reassured her that she did not have cancer and that she was going to be okay with more lessons and time.

In the weeks that followed, Elizabeth developed a love-hate relationship with her speaking valve, called a Passy Muir valve, which allowed her to speak when she breathed out and facilitated breathing through her mouth and nose rather than through the trach tube. She didn't like the feeling of the device on her throat and would try to take it out every chance she got.

One day when we were back at Shock Trauma for a follow-up exam, Elizabeth decided it was coming out, and her way.

Dr. Kirby, Elizabeth's new doctor, connected with Elizabeth right away. "Elizabeth needs a few more staples removed; we also want to check on how her damaged areas are healing," Dr. Kirby said.

After these procedures, I told the doctor how Elizabeth hated having to talk through the Passy Muir device connected to her trach tube and was always trying to adjust or remove the trach tube itself.

"Does she really need the trach opening still?" I asked. "I think she might be ready to breathe through her mouth."

Dr. Kirby looked from me to Elizabeth and said, "Let's see."

She released the band from around Elizabeth's neck that kept the trach tube in place. Before the doctor could take the tube out, Elizabeth took a deep breath and blew it out on her own.

"Can you breathe?" the doctor asked, and Elizabeth gave us two thumbs up. She had color in her face and a big smile to go with it.

Dr. Kirby started laughing, "This girl no doubt wanted that tube out," she said.

After a few minutes, there was a knock on the door, and in walked Elizabeth's brother, Logan. I knew he was coming to visit but not what time he would arrive. When Elizabeth saw Logan, she grabbed his hand and gestured for him to sit down next to her on the gurney. She showed him her throat without a trach tube and tried to speak to him but had some trouble getting the words out. The doctor told us that was to be expected and that in time she would relearn how to direct air flow through her mouth. I sat back in my chair watching Logan and Elizabeth talking with each other. The two most precious things in my life were there in that room with me.

~~~~~~~~~~~~~~

One day I went to do some laundry in the KKI laundry room, and when I returned, Elizabeth and her sitters were dancing. The sitters had turned on some music for her to listen to, they told me, but as soon as she heard it, she'd stood up on her own and started to dance, then waved them to come and join her. With each new move she did, the sitters and I clapped her on for more.

I wrote about this day in my journal and shared it on Caring Bridge with Elizabeth's friends and family. But when I got to the end of the journal and started to type my usual ending "Drive safely and please pay attention behind the wheel," my heart sank. In the past few weeks when Elizabeth wasn't doing well, I had been focusing on getting her better and had put the terrible secret I carried into the back of my mind. Typing those words brought it to the forefront again, and I questioned whether I should continue giving advice. I had been her distraction. Would people judge me?

With each journal entry I posted from then on, I struggled with guilt and shame and wondered if I should stop. Yet, as guilty as I felt, I did not want what had happened to Elizabeth to happen to her friends and their families. So, I kept silent.

~~~~~~~~~~~~~~

Elizabeth's discharge day from KKI approached, and she was scheduled for a follow-up appointment with her neurologists at the University of Maryland outpatient division for post Shock Trauma patients. The doctors were amazed at how well she was doing and asked me, to my great shock, if I wanted to take her home —they felt she was ready to go home and continue her rehab as an outpatient. They knew of a very good outpatient facility not far from where we lived and assured me that Elizabeth could receive the care she needed there.

"Can I take her now?" I asked eagerly. The doctors laughed at me and told me she would have to go through a few tests in the coming days, but if she passed them, she could go home. At this, Elizabeth screamed with joy.

"I am going to pass them, Mom, you wait and see," she said in her scratchy voice. As Elizabeth predicted, she did.

When the doctors gave us the green light for Elizabeth to come home, I called Jim and Frank to let them know the great news. Then, I wrote my final Caring Bridge journal entry.

Dear Friends,

Just wanted to say thank you to everyone for all your prayers and blessings to Elizabeth and her family. She is doing great, so great that she is coming home!! The doctors have cleared her to be released, and she will be home tomorrow. I want to thank everyone who took the time to write notes to Elizabeth and her family through this site. The notes were my lifeline; they were something I looked forward to at the end of a long day. I can't thank you enough for them. I would read them over and over sometimes when things were going bad for Elizabeth, and it would give me strength to continue on for her. Your words will be with me for the rest of my life. My only wish right now is that the friends and family (young and old) who have read my journals don't forget my message about being safe behind the wheel. Elizabeth is lucky, very lucky. She beat the odds and will one day get back to a normal life though, granted, it will be a long time in coming. But she does have a future, something many people who went through what she went through do not. Driving distracted is dangerous. Please do not let this journey happen to you or anyone in your family. Drive safely and pay attention behind the wheel!!! God bless you all!

Liz's Mom

Betty Shaw

CHAPTER 13

DEPRESSION

For the first few weeks after Elizabeth returned home, she was happy. Well-wishers knocked on our front door every day to visit her, and Elizabeth enjoyed all the attention and gifts. People who read my journal entries knew that UNO was her favorite game, so they brought her the game as a gift, and she played many rounds with her friends and family. Many nights, her friends came over to watch a movie in the living room. Elizabeth sometimes fell asleep during the movie, but no one seemed to mind. They all understood that she tired easily and stayed just to be there with her.

Elizabeth was regaining her appetite and finally putting back on some of the 30 pounds she'd lost. She never showed any signs of sadness so I never pursued setting up an appointment for her with a mental health therapist. This turned out to be a mistake, perhaps the biggest one I'd made yet.

With each session spent with her cognitive therapist, she became more aware of who she was and what had happened to her. She knew she had been in a car accident that she had caused. Her cognitive therapist advised me not to mention the accident or to answer any questions that she may have about it. Her friends and family were still coming by to see her, but the visits started to dwindle as the weeks passed.

Elizabeth's hair had only grown back to about an inch and a half in length, so the scars from her brain surgeries were still very visible on her head. Her good eye had healed very well, but the damage to her left eye showed prominently: a scar ran from the top of her forehead above her left eye diagonally down to her right eye socket. She had lost the muscle movement in her left eye lid and could open it only slightly. A large scar on her neck from her trach tube was still in its healing stages as well. None of our friends or family made any negative comments about her appearance, and the few times I took her out in public, people often came up to wish her well in her recovery, aware of her and her story from the newspapers.

Thanks to the positive reaction she was generally receiving from people, I didn't think twice about taking Elizabeth to a big shopping mall 45 minutes away from where we lived. I thought it would be fun for her to walk around and perhaps buy herself a treat.

As soon as we entered the mall, Elizabeth stopped and stood still in the middle of the busy walkway. "I remember these sounds," she said.

"What sounds?"

"The sounds of many people talking at one time, the sounds of shopping bags rubbing together and making a squeaky noise."

She looked up to the ceiling. "Oh, the sunlight coming through that window feels good on my skin."

I stood there watching her as she described what she was feeling and hearing. Then, she laughed and said, "Do you hear those kids crying? I remember that, too."

We both laughed and started to walk again. As we were walking, several people stared openly at Elizabeth, but luckily, she seemed unaware of them. As we walked farther into the mall, Elizabeth saw a kiosk station that sold hair extensions. She became excited and walked fast ahead of me toward it. My heart dropped. I knew she was going to ask if she could try some on and worried she would be refused because of the state of her hair.

I caught up with Elizabeth. As we walked closer to the woman at the extensions kiosk, she gestured for me to come try some on. Elizabeth asked the lady if she could try some on, too. The woman looked at Elizabeth's head and frowned, but then she noticed all the scars on her face. For a moment she was silent. She looked at me, then back at Elizabeth.

"Yes, you can. Sit down here, pretty lady, and let's see what we can do for you!" She smiled at Elizabeth, and Elizabeth smiled back. I breathed a silent sigh of relief. Elizabeth sat in the chair, and the woman began to put on the blonde hair extensions Elizabeth had requested. They did not fit her correctly, but she loved them, anyway. She swung her head back and forth, pretending that it was her own real hair.

At first, I stood back, watching Elizabeth enjoy her time with this kind-hearted woman. Then, I noticed two older women had stopped walking and were pointing at her. They were even laughing and whispering to each other. I stood there, unsure what to do. I thought about going up to those ignorant women and giving them a piece of my mind, but if I did, Elizabeth would want to know why. I just stood there, pain and sadness for Elizabeth piercing my body. Would this be the reaction she would have to deal with the rest of her life? To have been through so much to get where she was and then to have people laughing at her—that thought tortured me.

Elizabeth called me over to tell me how much she loved the hair and how much she missed her own hair. "My own hair," she said again.

I saw the change in her face and her attitude immediately. "I remember having my old hair," she said. "I used to put it up in a bun. My car accident took my hair away from me, didn't it, Mom?" I didn't answer her.

Then, she said, "It was my fault. I did this to myself." She started to pull the extensions from her head and then said firmly, "I'm done." She thanked the woman for letting her try the hair extensions on, turned to me, and said "I want to go home. Can you take me home now, please?"

We both left the mall that day in despair.

~~~~~~~~~~~~~~~

By the beginning of August, hardly any of Elizabeth's friends came to see her anymore. Most had graduated from high school that spring and were preparing to go to college. Others were about to resume high school or begin to work at a job. A few had even left the area to pursue their dreams. Everyone else seemed to be moving on with their lives, but Elizabeth wasn't. She still had a long road to recovery ahead of her. She couldn't drive; she couldn't work; and she had to learn how to read and write all over. The reality of this was setting in. Elizabeth still had one close friend, Kayla, but even she couldn't get Elizabeth to see that her situation was just temporary. By the middle of August, Elizabeth began to show signs of serious depression.

With each passing day, she sank deeper and deeper. She turned away the few friends who did stop by, telling them she wasn't feeling well or that she had to go somewhere with me. I knew she was lying to them, but I didn't know what to do. I thought it was just a phase, a part of her recovery, and that she would bounce back. I began to give her chores around the house so she could earn some spending money and get her mind off of her sorrows. But she struggled doing even the simplest of tasks and showed no interest in making money. She had no desire to watch TV and spent most of her time in her room.

Sometimes, she would draw or work on her cognitive homework, but most of the time she just lay on her bed and slept. When I knew she was not napping but it was quiet in her room, I would tiptoe up to her bedroom door and peek in. She had opened her closet door and was sitting on the floor, staring at herself in the mirror on the back of the door. She moved her hands over her head, feeling what little hair she had. Then, she moved her face closer to the mirror and examined each of her scars. As she moved her face back and forth in front of the mirror, I could hear sorrowful breaths coming from deep within her.

I missed the signs of Elizabeth's dangerous level of depression. Back then, labeling someone "depressed" was considered taboo. I felt alone in trying to figure out how to help Elizabeth and had no idea where to start.

It became a battle each day to get Elizabeth to attend her cognitive classes. She cried and begged me not to make her go, saying it made her think too much.

"I know the accident was my fault," she would lament, "and I made people sad because I got hurt." She told me that she felt really sorry for hurting her father and me and questioned why this happened.

"I was supposed to die; why didn't I?" she would ask. Questions like this were chilling reminders of my secret. Should I tell her it was my fault, too? Would that make her feel better? Would that make her sadness go away? I didn't know. The thought of telling her and the possibility that it would only make the situation worse kept me from getting the help we both needed.

The next day I attended Elizabeth's cognitive class with her. I wanted her to describe to the therapist what she had been feeling lately and had stressed the importance of telling the truth. The therapist asked me to leave the room so she and Elizabeth could talk alone. After 15 minutes, Elizabeth emerged from the room, and the therapist waved for me to come in.

"Elizabeth is seriously depressed," the therapist said. "Her situation needs to be addressed now, before it gets worse. I believe it would be beneficial for her to go someplace where she can get the care she needs. A mental hospital."

As she spoke, I was thinking, no way! I am *not* going to take my kid to a mental hospital. That's for crazy people, and my daughter is *not* crazy. I refused to believe that Elizabeth's emotional state was that bad. I had the mindset that once you went to a mental hospital, people would think you were nuts and would want nothing to do with you. I had definitely absorbed the stigma that so many people at that time held associated with mental health issues.

I thought perhaps Elizabeth just needed some medication to help her get through this phase of her recovery and in time she would work through her depression on her own. I thanked the therapist for her advice and took the paper with the hospital's contact information with me.

Once we got home, I called around trying to find a psychotherapist who could see Elizabeth as soon as possible, but each person I spoke to told me that there would be a wait of about two months. I couldn't believe it. After many calls, I was able to get an appointment for Elizabeth to be seen in a week—but the therapist did not take insurance, and I would have to pay in full. I'm sure being able to pay was the only reason I could get an appointment so fast; therapists are so expensive that many people simply can't afford them.

Thankfully, with Jim having been smart about money and having pre-pared for unforeseen tragic events, I was able to pay for this appointment. Moreover, the good insurance we had through his job helped lessen the stress that might have been put on our marriage had we also experienced financial difficulties. Instead, most of the medical bills that arrived in the daily mail were merely passed on to our insurance company for payment.

Meanwhile, I was so afraid Elizabeth might try to kill herself that I locked up everything she could use to hurt herself. I removed pills from medicine cabinets and locked them in the shed outside. I got rid of any rope and locked up all the eating or cooking knives in the house. From that day forward, I never left Elizabeth alone by herself. I was going to be "Supermom." Maybe that would be my ticket to forgiveness.

For the next several nights, after I gave Elizabeth her sleep medica-tion, I waited until she was asleep, put on one of my husband's old t-shirts with a front pocket, and kissed him goodnight. Then, slowly and silently, in order not to wake Elizabeth, I climbed into bed with her. I got as close to her as possible without disturbing her sleep and then reached into my shirt's front pocket and pulled out a shoestring removed from one of my husband's hockey skates. I tied one end around my wrist and the other end to Elizabeth's wrist. I thought that if she tried to get up and hurt herself, that shoestring would wake me up so I could stop her. We lay tied together all night long though I never really slept. I lay there for hours, praying to God to make Elizabeth happy again. I talked to my dad and to Julie, asking them to help me watch over Elizabeth. I asked God to stop torturing my daughter and to torture me instead.

Two days before Elizabeth's scheduled appointment with the therapist, I asked Elizabeth's friend Kayla to come over and spend a night with her, and Kayla agreed. I needed a night of good sleep and thought that maybe having a friend stay over would give Elizabeth something to look forward to. Maybe, also, she would share with Kayla what she was going through.

At first, the sleepover seemed to be going well. I could hear them in Elizabeth's bedroom listening to music and giggling. Thinking I was finally going to get a few hours of sleep that night, I climbed into bed and started to read a magazine. Just as I was starting to drift off, around 11:00 p.m. or so, I heard hurried footsteps and a knock at my door. It was Kayla.

"Something is wrong," she said. "It's Elizabeth."

I jumped out of bed and hurried to Elizabeth's bedroom. Elizabeth sat on the edge of her bed with her arms wrapped around herself like she was trying to hold herself. She rocked her body back and forth, her eyes glassy and red and a blank stare on her face.

I ran to her and began to shake her. "What is wrong?" I asked. "What is wrong?"

She snapped out of her fog then and started to talk. What I heard Elizabeth telling me next started my world crashing down once again.

"I don't want to live anymore," she said. "I hate the way I look. I feel like a freak. All my friends are off at college having fun, and what am I doing? I am at home relearning the fucking ABCs."

She didn't want to have the surgeries she knew were in her future, she said. She was afraid of the pain that followed each surgery. She couldn't shut her mind off, and every minute she was awake, she felt guilty, lonely, and left behind. She begged me to stop watching her every move and to leave her alone so she could stop the pain herself.

"You would be happier without me," she said. "I see you sad all the time, and I know it's because of me."

At that moment, I realized I could not fix my daughter on my own. I woke my husband and told him that I was taking Elizabeth to Dorchester General Hospital's mental health facility, Shore Behavioral Health. As I prepared to leave, both relief and guilt washed my body—I worried still that I was doing Elizabeth in, condemning her to a life of stigma and isolation.

The mental hospital was located just 20 minutes away. Once there, I turned off the engine, leaned over to Elizabeth, and gave her a hug.

"We're here to get you medication and therapy to help you feel better," I told her. "Your dad and I and your friends love you so much. We just want you to be happy again. I think this is the place to make that happen for you."

Elizabeth began to cry. "I can't," she said. "Life is just too hard. I feel sad and lonely all the time. These feelings are with me every minute of every day. I don't know how to make them stop."

Then, her voice rose to a shriek. "The accident was my fault, and I don't deserve to live," she cried. "God should have saved someone else. I think you would be happier without me, and if I were gone, nobody would have to worry about me anymore."

I found myself begging for her to stay here on earth with me once again. This time, it was not in a trauma room; it was in my car in front of a mental hospital, getting ready to take Elizabeth into an unknown world. The same words I had spoken to her just four months earlier when she was flown to Shock Trauma, clinging to life, spilled out from deep within me. I reached over and held on to her. She wrapped her hands around my body and put her head under my chin. I felt her arms, her head, and the sorrow coming from deep within her soul. I squeezed her even tighter.

CHAPTER 14

DOUBLE DOORS

After checking in at the front desk and explaining Elizabeth's mental state, I learned that I needed to register her. After completing that process, we were both escorted to a room in the emergency area of the hospital. There Elizabeth changed into a gown, and a lab tech drew blood to check for illicit drugs and for pregnancy.

While awaiting the results of the blood work, I called Frank, who showed up in less than an hour, just as the emergency room doctor for the evening came by to talk to Elizabeth. The doctor informed us that the tests had turned out negative, and then he asked Elizabeth some questions, beginning with, "Do you have a plan?"

"What do you mean?" Elizabeth responded, puzzled.

"How do you plan on taking your life?"

The room went quiet. I could feel my heart beating inside my chest, waiting for Elizabeth's answer.

"I don't have a plan," Elizabeth said finally. "I just want these sad feelings inside of me to stop."

After 20 more minutes of questions about Elizabeth's accident and medications, the doctor informed Frank and me that two other doctors, one a physician and the other a psychologist, both certified in mental health disorders, would be arriving soon to evaluate Elizabeth and determine whether she should be admitted. Frank, Elizabeth, and I waited another two hours before they arrived. While waiting, Frank and I just held Elizabeth's hands and reassured her that things would get better for her.

When the two doctors arrived, they introduced themselves. Then, they asked Elizabeth about her car accident, and the psychologist asked her the same question that the ER doctor had posed: "Do you have a plan?"

This time, before answering Elizabeth looked at me. Then, she replied, "No."

The doctors noticed Elizabeth's eye contact with me and took her to a more private room so she could continue the conservation without us in the room. Frank and I each gave her a kiss, and then we found ourselves alone. He and I just sat there in that bright, cold, empty room, not saying a word to each other. He sighed in frustration and shook his head back and forth in my direction.

Half an hour later, Elizabeth and the doctors returned to the cubicle, and Elizabeth clambered into a hospital bed where someone would watch over her. Frank and I followed the doctors to a small private room where another woman wearing a white jacket and holding a clipboard waited for us.

"Your daughter's mental condition is critical," the psychologist told us. "She is choosing life right now but only because of you, her mother. She worries about the sadness you will feel once she is gone."

Both doctors agreed that Elizabeth's depression and feelings of hopelessness would grow stronger each day and that it was only a matter of time before her desire for the pain to stop would win out. Once I told them about sleeping with Elizabeth at night and tying a shoestring on each of our wrists to prevent her from hurting herself, the meeting came to an abrupt end. The doctors decided to admit Elizabeth immediately.

Frank could not believe it. "Why haven't you told me about all the this?" he snapped at me.

He was right. I should have asked him for help, but I still felt that the responsibility to put our lives back together was mine and mine alone.

Because Elizabeth was over 18, we, her parents, could not grant permission for her to be admitted, but the doctors had the legal right to do so, based on their assessment of her mental health. They then admitted Elizabeth involuntarily so she couldn't check herself out. This also meant Frank and I no longer had any say in her care. Our daughter was in the custody of a state mental hospital.

I felt relief. The burden of keeping my daughter alive was now on someone else's shoulders. Frank didn't say anything. He just listened, then once the meeting finished, went back to our daughter's side.

Elizabeth apologized for all the trouble she had caused us and again begged us just to let her die. We both held her hands and told her how much we loved her and felt so lucky and happy to have her in our lives. Hours went by, and the night turned into the morning. Finally, a nurse from the mental health facility side of the hospital came to take Elizabeth to her room. Time for Elizabeth to be properly admitted to the psych ward! We could not go with her. We both gave her a kiss goodbye. Then, they wheeled Elizabeth away.

As I walked to my car with Elizabeth's father, he gave me an earful, and I just listened, saying nothing. After he finished, I drove to the closest convenience store and bought a fresh pack of cigarettes. I drove myself to an abandoned shopping mall parking lot, got out of the car, and smoked one cigarette after another. With each new cigarette I lit, my mind spun further and further out of control.

~~~~~~~~~~~~~~~

Dealing with loved ones who suffer from depression really hurts, serving up loads of loneliness, frustration, and a sense of inadequacy, stirred together, making you yourself feel not good enough. Why are they so unhappy? What am I doing wrong? Do they not love me enough to want to live? Then, the feelings of anger set in because you don't understand. Depression is usually accompanied by other conditions, like anxiety, bipolar disorder, and obsessive-compulsive disorder. Each person experiences depression in a unique way. Yet, a common thread sews all depressed people together: uncontrollable feelings of despair and sadness. Getting up each day to do the simplest task represents a physical and mentally challenging ordeal, a drain on body and soul. It is an illness, a disease, just like cancer, but unfortunately, unlike cancer, very little help exists for those suffering from depression. Our mental health system is inadequate and underfunded. We need more facilities and additional research on depression and other mental conditions.

~~~~~~~~~~~~~~~

When I returned the next day to visit Elizabeth in the mental hospital, I encountered the conditions I had feared. The youngest patient there, Elizabeth was surrounded by patients with severe drug and alcohol addiction issues who would scream at the staff to give them a sip of liquor. Elizabeth showed me her room and told me about her roommate, an older woman who didn't speak a word to Elizabeth. There were no locks on the doors, and at night, Elizabeth said, the other patients screamed and cried. She had a hard time sleeping out of fear that another patient would come into her room and hurt her. How could she possibly get the help she needed being in a place like that? But this was all that was available. She was in the custody of the state now, and there was nothing I could do.

In the days that followed, Elizabeth responded well to her medications though, at least according to the doctors, who said she showed signs of improvement. At last, something positive! Her one-on-one therapy sessions seemed to help her as well, but the group therapy sessions did not. She had to listen to many stories of how the other residents had become drug addicts or alcoholics, and those stories made her sad. This infuriated me. I did not understand how hearing these stories could possibly help Elizabeth, and I repeatedly butted heads with her counselor. I was told these sessions were mandatory.

Elizabeth's condition improved gradually. I still feared for her safety and emphatically let the staff know my feelings on this issue. Needless to say, neither the staff nor the counselor liked me much, but I didn't care. Elizabeth's safety concerned me more.

Visiting hours at the mental hospital lasted from noon to 2:00 p.m. and from 5:00 p.m. to 7:00 p.m. I would visit Elizabeth at both times every day. We played lots of UNO and board games, and I even brought my mom and sisters with me to visit. Jim and Frank came every evening with me as well. One day, Kayla and her mom came to visit, too, but Elizabeth asked that we not tell any of her other friends.

Each day, I brought Elizabeth a letter from either me or Jim. I would tell her not to read the letter then but to save it for when our visit was over so she would have a little something to look forward to. They were just little notes of how proud we were of her and that we couldn't wait for her to come home. I would tell her about her cat Amy, how she slept every night on her pillow, meowing for Elizabeth to come home. Jim wrote about his day at work or the weather.

Sometimes, Elizabeth would write a letter for me, Frank, or Jim in return. They were simple, sweet letters, telling us how much she loved us and that she was feeling better and not having those bad thoughts as much.

Once, she wrote a letter to herself, on a pink piece of construction paper. She wrote about why she was there and that she had not felt like killing herself and that was a good thing. In another letter, she drew a smiley face and ended by writing, "I hope tomorrow will be better," followed by "THANK YOU, GOD!" She drew little hearts across the piece of paper.

Looking back, I believe that letter marked the beginning of Elizabeth's long road to recovery and to forgiving herself.

~~~~~~~~~~~~~~~

By the fifth day of Elizabeth's stay at the mental hospital, I was showing signs of exhaustion. I wasn't sleeping, I wasn't eating much, and all I did was worry about what Elizabeth was doing and if she was safe.

One afternoon when visiting time with Elizabeth ended and we had to say our goodbyes, we walked to the double door exit together while a staff member followed behind us as usual. We kissed and hugged each other. Then, Elizabeth started to get upset. She wanted to come home with me. In a hurry, the staff member shooed me out. I gave Elizabeth one more kiss goodbye and walked through the double doors. I turned around as the doors were closing, and I heard Elizabeth ask the staff member if she could give me one more kiss goodbye. The staff member said no. Then, I heard my little girl crying, really crying, the kind of cry that breaks your heart. The doors had fully closed by then. I tried to open them, but they had locked. I just stood there at those double doors, listening to Elizabeth's cries, muffled by the wood between us. I put my ear to the door and heard her cries fading as she walked away.

It was then that my cell phone rang, the one I had used to text Elizabeth on that horrible day. I took the cell phone out of my pocket, but I didn't answer it. I just held it in my hand. This phone has destroyed my life! I screamed inside my head. Because I was an irresponsible mother, I could not even give my daughter that one more kiss goodbye. Because I was an irresponsible mother, she was locked up in a mental hospital.

As I sat in my car getting ready to leave, I finally broke down. All the emotions that I had been keeping bottled up inside me came bursting out. I cried for my daughter, Julie. I cried for my daughter, Elizabeth. I cried for myself. I wanted so badly for my dad to be there with me. I longed for his arms to hold me and tell me that taking his granddaughter here was the right thing to do and that everything would be fine. I had sunk to the lowest point of my life.

~~~~~~~~~~~~~~~

The doctors released Elizabeth on her ninth day at the mental hospital. When Frank and I came to get her, we were directed to a small meeting room inside the area where our daughter was staying and just off to the side from those dreaded exit double doors. The counselor went over the progress that Elizabeth had made during her stay and gave us information and contacts for her continued care as an outpatient. Elizabeth would be seeing a therapist on a weekly basis and a psychiatrist two weeks after her release and monthly thereafter to monitor her and make any necessary adjustments to her medications.

Toward the end of that meeting, the counselor looked at me.

"You're Elizabeth's primary caregiver?"

"Yes."

"Then I highly suggest you seek counseling for yourself, too. Caring for someone with depression issues is physically and mentally draining to the caregiver as well. You need to be healthy for Elizabeth's sake."

This was a new idea. I had been so consumed with Elizabeth's mental health that I had never considered nurturing my own.

Once the meeting was over, we emerged to find Elizabeth standing in front of the exit double doors. She held a brown paper bag containing all of her belongings, and she wore a smile that I hadn't seen since she was a little girl.

"Mommy and Daddy," she cried. "Take me home!"

CHAPTER 15
CALL ME LIZ

Elizabeth was not cured; she had just stabilized. We still needed to keep a close eye on her behavior to watch for any signs of her becoming depressed again and to get her help swiftly. I went back to sleeping in bed with Elizabeth each night, but this time she knew about it. It was now something we both looked forward to. We would talk about simple things: what she wanted to buy with the money she earned from doing her chores, what makeup she would wear again, and other things of everyday life. Once she was asleep, I would watch and listen to her breathing and draw as close to her as I could without waking her so I could feel her warm body next to mine. Jim would check in on us sometimes, and I could see he missed me sleeping with him.

Just like before, after being released from the brain rehab center, Elizabeth enjoyed being home again. Happy at first, as the weeks passed, she became argumentative, blunt, and bold when she talked to me. We would have arguments over the dumbest things. What few friends she had left came over to the house less and less frequently. They had a hard time dealing with the immature way in which Elizabeth now spoke and acted and the way in which she would make inappropriate comments she found funny then get confused when others didn't laugh. Elizabeth would say whatever was on her mind and not realize the impact of her words. It broke my heart to see Elizabeth have these embarrassing moments. I would try to correct her, but she got defensive and mad at me for trying to reteach her proper social skills. The doctors told us that damage to her frontal lobe, the "executive center" of the brain, erased her social skills and diminished self-control. Her short-term memory as well was impaired.

In other ways, too, Elizabeth had changed. She used to like rap, but after her accident, her tastes switched to pop music. Before the accident, she liked white chocolate, but after the accident she preferred milk chocolate. She used to eat junk food rarely but now she couldn't get enough of it. At first, I gave in and let her have whatever she wanted, but when she started to put on weight, I limited her junk food. She couldn't sit still long enough to watch a TV show, let alone a movie. She used to dress in flashy clothes with pretty colors, but now she wore oversized plain-colored clothes, perhaps to hide the newly gained pounds. She still enjoyed playing UNO, but now if her game partner was winning, she would get upset and insist on playing the game over and over until she won.

One day, after another silly argument over something trivial, she screamed at me, "Stop calling me Elizabeth! I am not her anymore. She is gone, and she is never coming back. Call me Liz from now on."

I stood there confused at first, but then I realized she was right: She really was not the Elizabeth I had known from before the car accident. That Elizabeth died on April 7, 2012. She was gone and was never coming back. In front of me now was a scared, lonely, and confused young girl who was starting her life over again.

In the days after Liz told me that she no longer was Elizabeth, I fell into an even deeper depression. In my mind, I had failed as a mother because both my daughters had died—maybe Frank and I shouldn't have consented to giving Julie the steroid shot. Even though Liz was still here on earth with me, I was grieving the loss of Elizabeth and Julie as well. I tried to hide my depression from everyone, but Jim noticed and finally intervened.

One night as I was brushing my teeth and getting ready to go get into bed with Liz, Jim took my hand.

"What's wrong?"

"I can't explain it," I said. "I just feel like this is all my fault."

"But it's not."

It was time to tell him. "It was me Liz was texting that day."

"I know, Betty."

"You do?"

He nodded. "I just put two and two together. It had to be somebody, and, unfortunately, it ended up being you."

I began to cry, and he pulled me close. He didn't judge me, and he wasn't upset with me.

"But I need you to get help," he said. "You can't continue on this way."

I promised I would.

On the drive to my first appointment, I asked myself, what good is this going to do? I already felt overwhelmed with stress—I just didn't have time for this. I told myself I was just going to sit there and listen to what the therapist had to say to me and be done with it.

The therapist's name was Neil. In his early 60s, he wore a grayish sweater vest with a nicely manicured beard.

After Neil and I introduced ourselves, he examined the forms I had filled out about my history, then looked at me and said, "You have been through hell and back, haven't you?"

I just burst into tears and started talking. Just an hour before, I'd been mad at my husband for making me come. Now, here I was, spilling my guts to a total stranger. As I continued to tell him about the nightmare my life had been since the accident, he handed me a box of tissues.

"Don't stop," he said. "Get it all out."

I took a deep breath and told him my secret. After I'd finished describing how my text had caused Liz's accident, I stopped talking and waited for the look of reproach to appear on his face. I waited several seconds for it to come, but it never did. He looked at me in puzzlement instead and then said, while shaking his head, "What, you think you're the first mother to make a mistake with her child?" Then, he gave me this big smile.

I was speechless at first. Then, a big, long forgotten laugh came out of me. To think I would never make a mistake in raising my child was a foolish way to think. I could feel the burden of my secret being released from my soul. He told me it was time to stop blaming myself, that my daughter had been 17 at that time and most likely knew texting and driving was wrong but chose not to listen. For whatever reason, she was one of the unfortunate people who had to pay the price for driving distracted.

I never missed a session with Neil from that day on. He was like a wise old grandfather, whom I trusted completely. He always wore a sweater vest, even on warm days, which I found comforting; it was his trademark. With each session I attended, I felt my old self coming back. I still felt remorse for my mistake in texting Liz, but the guilt I carried slowly began to fade.

Chapter 16
STARTING TO TELL

Elizabeth's struggles continued. She could not work or drive.

Other than her twice-weekly cognitive classes and therapy sessions now every other week, Elizabeth had a lot of time on her hands. She felt lonely and left out of life.

Bowling helped her to escape some of her loneliness. She developed a strong love for this sport. Although we bowled a lot together, at times Liz wanted to bowl without us. Those times she would reach out to her old friends on Facebook to join her at the bowling alley. Unfortunately, they were often too busy with college, jobs, and life to do so. Some who responded said they had other things to do or "maybe another time." She hung on to the latter responses as a glimmer of hope and would bug those persons over and over until no more responses came.

In general, Liz was trying to reconnect with her old friends. Looking at other old friends' Facebook pages and seeing everyone getting together and having fun made matters worse. One day, I read her Facebook page and burst into tears after reading her plaintive plea, "Can anyone hang out with me? I have no friends."

One day, I dropped Liz off to go bowling by herself. I asked if I could bowl with her, but she said in an angry voice, "I would look stupid bowling with my mom!"

I accepted the tone without comment. I knew the source. Earlier, on Facebook, she had again sought friends to go bowling with her, and not one person had responded. On the way to the bowling alley, she did not speak. From her lowered head, I could both see and feel her sadness.

Before Liz exited the car, I made one more try: "Liz, I would love to bowl with you."

She slammed the car door, leaving without a word. I watched her enter the bowling alley, knowing that she would be bowling all by herself. I pictured other bowlers there, laughing and having fun and worried that Liz would be asking herself questions like:

"Why doesn't anyone want to hang out with me?"

"Is my face too ugly to look at?"

"What's wrong with me?"

I had to force myself not to just show up and bowl with her, anyway. Tears were streaming down my face and that would have made things worse. Liz blames herself for my tears.

During this time, whenever Liz saw family members or neighbors we would run into when walking around our neighborhood to get some fresh air and exercise, she would tell them everything was fine and that she was doing great.

"Why do you do that?" I asked finally.

"I don't know," she said. "I guess I don't want them to pity me."

She and Kayla still got together occasionally, though. One time, the two of them went out together, and Liz came back looking flushed and excited.

"What did you all do?" I asked.

"Oh, just walked around Target. I pretended to be a retard chasing after Kayla. We cracked up as people at the store stared at us."

I became furious with Liz. "That's so cruel," I said. "You can't make fun of people with disabilities like that. Of all people, you should know that. How dare you do such a thing!" I yelled.

"It was no big deal," she said, "and you have no right to be yelling at me!"

"But why," I asked, a bit more calmly. "Why did you do that?"

I stood there waiting for her to answer me, and after a few huffs and puffs of attitude, the real reason came out.

"I feel bad for what I did to myself," she said. "The accident was my fault, and I am the one who made my face like this. I wanted people to laugh with me, not at me." Then, she started to cry. Through her tears she said, "I am blind in my left eye, I can't hear out of my left ear, and I have this huge scar that runs across my face. You don't know what it is like to have people staring at you because of the way you look."

I stood there shocked but realized she was right. I *didn't* know what it was like for her. I didn't see Liz's scars and disfigured face any more when I looked at her. Like any parent would, I only saw my lovely young daughter.

I reached for Liz and held her in my arms. I told her she was beautiful and that her scars would fade in time. I let her cry for a while before I told her to promise me she would *never* do such a thing like that again. She nodded emphatically.

"Maybe my next surgery will make me prettier," she said.

Liz was scheduled for another reconstructive surgery with Dr. Dorafshar in December 2012 because the titanium plates and screws in her head had come to the surface of her skin. For Liz, this meant the fear and uncertainty of the surgery and knowing the pain that came afterward. She wanted the surgery to be over, so she did not tell her doctor how depressed she felt because of the way she looked.

At the consultation appointment before her surgery, when Liz was out of the room talking to the nurses, I filled Dr. Dorafshar in about her struggles. I told him that she was upset by the scar that ran across her face and how she would cover up the scar from her trach with ridiculously large necklaces. I told him to do whatever he could to help my daughter feel better about her appearance.

In the days before the surgery, Liz became moody and fragile, but the reconstructive surgery went well. Not only did Dr. Dorafshar do what was needed, but after my request, he also slipped in a few extra procedures to improve the appearance of Liz's face. It took weeks for the swelling to go down, but the difference in Liz's appearance was significant. The scar that ran across her face and her tracheotomy scar were reduced to half their previous sizes, and these two changes put a new smile on Liz's face. With the help of a little makeup and a new hairdo thanks to her Aunt Lisa who owns a hair salon, Liz started to feel better about the way she looked. She knew she had more surgeries ahead of her, but seeing the positive results from this one made her less anxious about the future.

I had stopped taking Liz with me when I ran errands after our horrible experience at the shopping mall, but now I started again. When she and I went out in public, people still stared, and this time she knew it. Though she never said anything to me about it, I could see the hurt and pain it caused her. I would try and get her mind off this by handing her $20 and telling her to go buy something fun, and off she would beeline toward the makeup counter. Then, I would notice a salesperson staring at her, prompting me to run over and say abrasively, "Do you have a problem? Why are you staring at my daughter?"

Not everyone would stare at Liz; some people who knew of her situation would come up and ask her how she was doing. It was around this time when Liz first started to be honest with others and tell them the truth. She began to tell people that she had been in a car accident because she was texting. She would tell some details about her accident, but most of what she said was inaccurate and confusing to understand. She would end by saying, "Please, don't use your phone when you are driving; don't be like me."

The first time she said this, I panicked. I worried they would ask Liz whom she was texting. But so far no one had. My secret was still safe, but I knew it wouldn't be for long. One day she was going to make the connection that someone else had to be on the other end. My day of telling Liz would have to come soon.

Photos

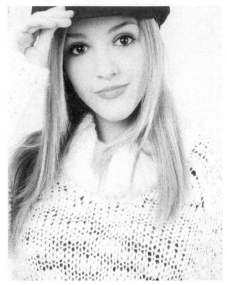

Liz's Barbizon School of Modeling head shot, taken in 2010 when she was in 10th grade. (Courtesy of Betty Shaw)

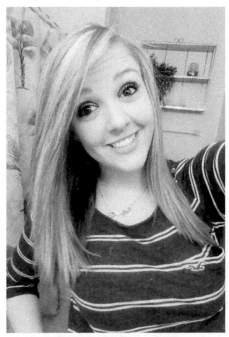

A selfie Liz took of herself during her senior year of high school. (Courtesy of Betty Shaw)

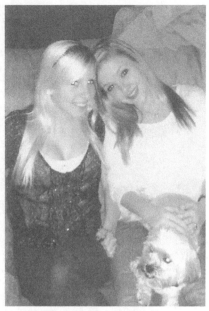

Liz (right) and her friend Kayla Haley the night before the accident. In less than 24 hours, Liz's life would be forever changed. (Courtesy of Betty Shaw)

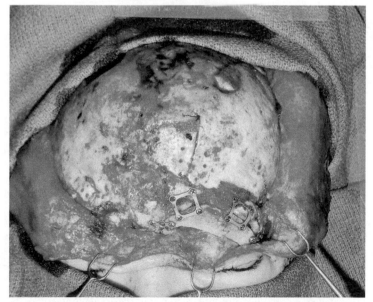

Graphic picture of Liz's skull taken by medical staff during her 11-hour facial reconstruction surgery. (Courtesy of Dr. Amir Dorafshar)

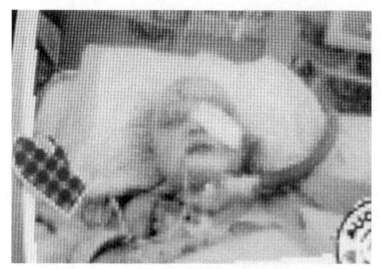

Liz, bandaged and battered, in the ICU, 10 days after her accident.
(Courtesy of Betty Shaw)

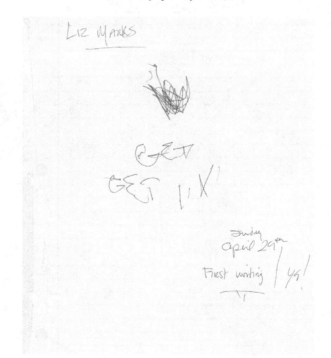

Liz's first communication three weeks after the accident, "Get it,"
signifying that she understood what Betty said to her.
(Courtesy of Betty Shaw)

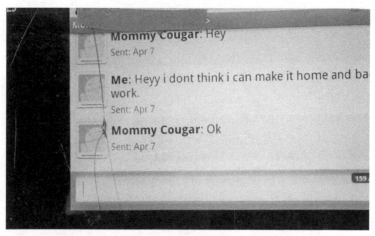

The exchange of texts between Liz and Betty which caused the accident.
(Courtesy of Betty Shaw)

Mommy Cougar: Hey
Sent: Apr 7

Me: Heyy i dont think i can make it home and ba
work.
Sent: Apr 7

Mommy Cougar: Ok
Sent: Apr 7

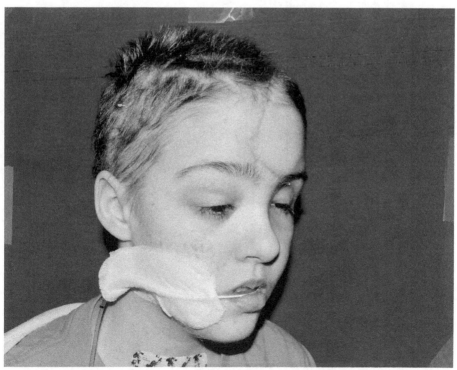

Liz, a month after the accident, fighting an infection which rendered her weak and required several antibiotics. (Courtesy of Dr. Amir Dorafshar)

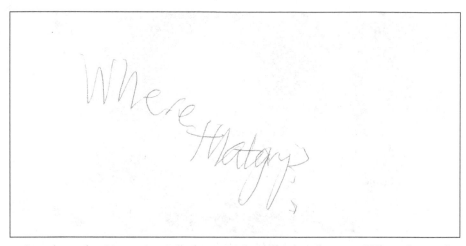

Betty knew that Liz was regaining her cognitive skills when she wrote "Where that guy" (Where's that guy?) after spotting a handsome male nurse, whom the female nurses nicknamed "Nurse Cupcake," in the hallway of the hospital. (Courtesy of Betty Shaw)

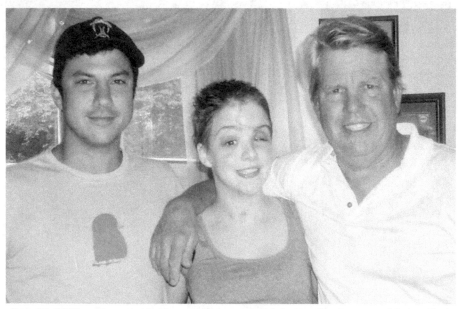

June 21, 2012 — Homecoming Day. Liz, pictured with her brother Logan and father, back home for the first time, two and a half months after the accident. (Courtesy of Betty Shaw)

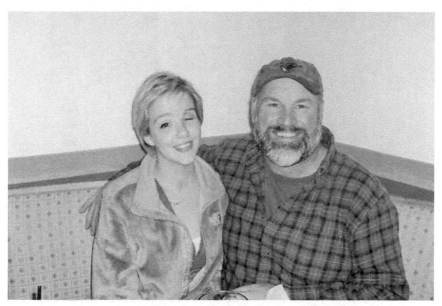

Liz and Robert Horton. Working nearby, Robert rushed to the scene when he heard the crash and helped keep Liz alive until emergency personnel arrived.
(Courtesy of Betty Shaw)

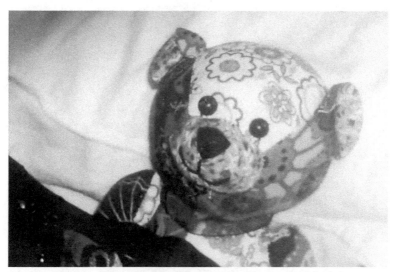

Liz slept with this teddy bear, made by her Aunt Trudy when she was a young girl. "Julie Bear" symbolized the bond between Liz and the twin sister that she lost at birth. (Courtesy of Betty Shaw)

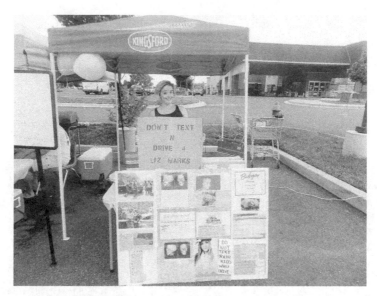

*Liz, at a grocery store in her hometown, attending one of
her first events in 2013 and proudly displaying her campaign motto.
(Courtesy of Betty Shaw)*

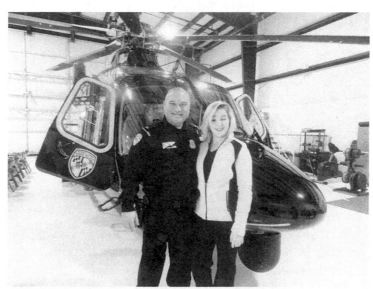

*Liz with paramedic Jeremy Krebs, who kept her alive on the medevac
flight to Shock Trauma in Baltimore. (Courtesy of Betty Shaw)*

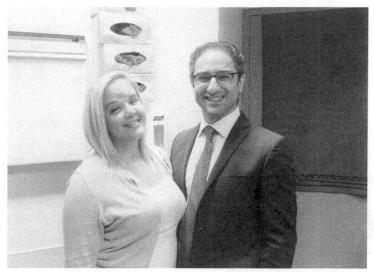

Liz and her esteemed plastic surgeon, Dr. Amir Dorafshar, in his office at Johns Hopkins Hospital. (Courtesy of Dr. Amir Dorafshar) Currently Dr. Dorafshar is Chief of Plastic Surgery at Rush University Medical Center in Chicago.

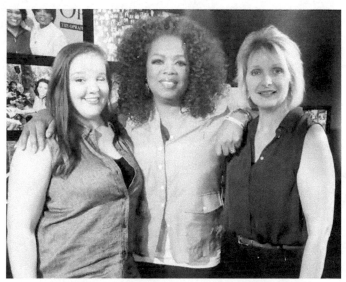

Liz and Betty flank Oprah Winfrey, after appearing on her Where Are They Now? show in August 2015. (Courtesy of OWN).

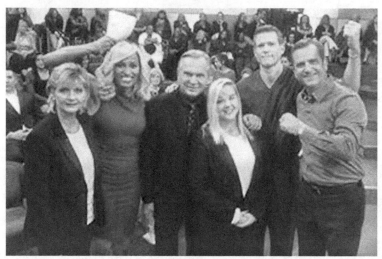

Betty and Liz, surrounded by the hosts of The Doctors
after they appeared on their show in November 2014

Part Three

TRIUMPH

"The human spirit needs to accomplish, to achieve, to triumph, to be happy."

Ben Stein

Betty Shaw

CHAPTER 17
ANGEL AT WALMART

Liz still spent most of her time alone. Bowling remained her escape, and a few times a week she would bowl with the guy who worked at the bowling alley, a nice young man named John, on whom Liz had developed a crush. One day, though, when I came to pick up Liz, she was quiet and didn't have the normal post-bowling smile on her face.

"What's wrong?"

"Nothing. I am fine, Mom!"

We didn't speak a word to each other the rest of the drive home. When we got home, Liz went straight to her room and shut the door. She knew I didn't like her door being shut so I knocked on the door and asked her to leave it ajar.

"Why?" she snapped back. "So, I don't kill myself?"

"What, is that what you want to do now, hurt yourself?" I said back, trying not to panic. "Do I have to take you back to the mental hospital again? What happened to make you feel this way again, what went wrong today?"

I waited for her to scream back, but she didn't. She sat on her bed with her head down and said softly, "He doesn't like me."

She had told John that she liked him—a thing she never would have done before her accident when she always played it cool around her crushes—and asked him if he liked her back. But, sadly, he'd replied with, "No, I like you just as a friend."

I sat down next to Liz, put my arms around her, and said I was sorry. I was sorry for yelling at her, and I was sorry that a boy she liked didn't like her back. We spent an hour just lying in her bed. Once she stopped crying, I started to share my heartfelt stories with her from when I was a young girl. I put a funny spin on them, and it seemed to help her feel better.

Then, she asked me, "Why did God save my life? Why didn't He just let me die so I wouldn't have to go through all this sadness?"

I asked her, "Are you talking about the sadness because the boy doesn't like you or the sadness of what you have been through?"

She said, "Both. But really, Mom, why didn't I die?"

I told her I didn't know why, that it was something that she was going to have to figure out on her own. It was the first truly deep and honest conversation we'd had since her accident.

Before we finished, I asked her, "Do you want to hurt yourself?"

"I guess not," she said. "It just felt good to get it out of my body and just scream the words out loud." She promised me that if she started to feel sad again, she would tell me.

We stood up, and I put my arms on Liz's shoulders, looked straight into her eyes, and said with conviction, "God left you here on this earth for a reason, and one day you will know that reason. I love you."

I started to walk out of her room, but before I left, she said, "I love you, too, Mom. Thanks."

~~~~~~~~~~~~~~

One cold, overcast day in late December, about a week before Christmas, Liz and I went to our local Walmart to drop off yet another new prescription at the pharmacy. Liz's brain was regenerating itself so her dosage and type of medicine changed quite often. As we stood in line to drop off the prescription, people began to stare at Liz. Once I reached the window, I quickly gave the clerk the prescription slip, along with the information she requested. I started to leave, telling the clerk we would pick it up later when she told me it would only take a few minutes and that we could wait if we liked. I hesitated for a second, but Liz jumped in and said, "Yes."

As we stood there waiting, I noticed one woman blatantly staring at Liz. An attractive, nicely-dressed, middle-aged woman with short dark hair in the line in front of the pharmacy pick-up area, she looked at Liz and then turned away, but a few seconds later, her eyes fixated on Liz again. Then, she did the head-to-toe stare, the type of stare that brought my blood to a boil.

The protective part of me came bursting out, and I headed right for this woman. But as I started to walk up to her, I felt a hand grabbing my upper arm. I stopped in my tracks and turned to see who was stopping me from pouncing on Liz's attacker. It was Liz.

"Let me go talk to this woman; you stay here," she said. Then she whispered firmly, "You embarrass me when you do it."

Before I could respond, Liz walked up to the monstrous woman who had been staring at her. I stood back waiting for my opportunity to come swooping in and rip this lady to shreds. I pictured how I would hurt her like in the movie, *The Revenant,* where a rogue mother bear tore Leonardo DiCaprio's character to pieces. That was going to be me if Liz came back to me crying.

Liz began to talk. At first, the woman reacted the same way that most people would when I approached them—she looked shocked and angry. But as Liz continued to describe what had happened to her, the woman's face changed. She was totally focused on what Liz was saying. Her body melted from a defensive stance to a more relaxed posture. Her eyes started to tear up, and she swallowed and swallowed like she was preventing herself from bursting into a big cry.

Liz finished and began to walk away, but the woman, a total stranger to my daughter, then put her arms around Liz and gave her a big, loving hug.

"You are a beautiful, brave young woman," the woman said.

She then asked Liz if she was on Facebook because she wanted to be friends with her. Then, she said the magic words that would change Liz's life: "Can you come to my son's school and share your story?"

Chapter 18
A REASON FOR LIVING

A week later, Liz and I passed a rainy afternoon playing UNO, her cognitive homework spread out on the kitchen table. Liz idly picked up her homework, then turned to me and said, "I think I know why God wanted me to live."

By then, I had started to cook dinner and turned to her from the stove, thinking she was going to say she wanted to raise kittens or save whales. "You do? Well, that is great."

"He saved me so I could save lives," she said. I stood there, shocked. She continued by telling me that she wanted to do what the lady at Walmart said she should do—go to schools to tell her story. She said she felt good about herself after telling people what had happened to her and that maybe her story would save other people from texting and driving.

I walked over to her and got down on my knees to get closer to her. I told her how proud I was to have her as my daughter.

"Mom, can you help me?"

Well, let me tell you, if I had had on a Wonder Woman outfit underneath my clothes and there had been a phone booth nearby, I would have jumped into that booth, spun around, and exited the booth, revealing my true identity, hands on my hips, exclaiming, "Yes! Yes, I can!" Instead, I held back my tears of joy.

"I will do whatever I can to help you," I promised. "When you are finished with your schoolwork, write down some ideas of what you want to do."

She gave me a big hug and went back to her work. She was still at the kitchen table when I slipped away and went to my bathroom. I got down on my knees, put my hands together, and thanked God for sending that angel to us in Walmart.

~~~~~~~~~~~~~~~

My fantasies of being Supermom faded with each day as the reality of what Liz asked me to do triggered nagging concerns. The more I thought about it, the more I wasn't sure if it was a good idea. How could I let her get up on stage by herself with hundreds of students looking directly at her? What if one of them made a smart remark or laughed at her, like the two women had done at the mall? Would Liz go back to being depressed and have thoughts of suicide again? I didn't know what to do.

On top of all this, I knew I still had to tell her who was on the other end of her text conversation. Would telling her it was me jeopardize her mental health? I constantly prayed to God, asking Him to help me. In my prayers, I would always ask over and over, "God, please tell me what to do. Give me a sign. I need a sign from You, please."

One day, I was ironing my husband's work clothes. I like to iron; it's a way for me to relax and not think about anything. This time, though, while standing over the ironing board, I couldn't get my mind off of what to do about Liz wanting to share her story. I turned on the TV and didn't change the channel. The screen snapped to the middle of a movie called *Seven Pounds*, in which Will Smith plays a character named Ben, who seemed to know he was dying. For whatever reason, he was meeting people who needed transplants of certain organs in order to continue living. I didn't understand the story and really didn't pay much attention to it. I just kept ironing and wondering what I should do about Liz when I heard a 911 operator in the movie asking Ben, "What is the emergency?" By this time, Ben was sitting in a bathtub filled with ice.

He told the 911 operator, "There has been a suicide."

The operator asked, "Who is the victim?"

Ben answered, "Me."

As Ben was sitting in that bathtub dying, scenes from his life flashed before him. One of his final visions was of him using his cell phone when he was driving. His fiancée was sitting in the front passenger seat of the car, and he was looking down at his cell phone. In one second, his life changed forever—he crashed his car, and the love of his life died because he was driving distracted. He killed himself in order to donate his organs to the people he'd met; his guilt was simply too much for him to live with.

I was so focused on the movie that I didn't realize I was burning my husband's shirt until I smelled the fabric burning. I quickly lifted up the iron, placed it on the kitchen counter, looked toward the ceiling, and told God, "Thank you. Thank you for my sign!"

The next day, I sat Liz down at the kitchen table. In my hand, I held her old cell phone.

"I have something to tell you," I began, "and I might cry after I tell you."

She looked at me, confused.

"I know who you were texting when you had your accident— "

"Who?" she interrupted.

I looked straight into her eyes and said, "It was me."

"*You*?"

"Yes. Me." I pulled up the text conversation we were having with each other on her phone and showed her the text message that she was reading when she had her car accident, the one that contained just two letters: "OK." She held the phone in her hands for a few seconds, then sat there in silence. I waited for her to look up and shout at me about how it was me who ruined her life and took away her dreams of becoming a model and made her lose all her friends.

She lifted her head. Here it was, the moment I had been dreading.

"I lied to you, Mom," she said. "I used my cell phone when I was driving all the time. Everyone else was doing it so I thought it was okay. I'm so sorry."

I couldn't believe what I was hearing. I had been ready to beg for her forgiveness and tell her how sorry I was for what I had done to her, but instead *she* was the one who was apologizing to me. I just hugged her and started to cry. I don't know what we said to each other then, but I remember feeling a sense of total relief. The burden of keeping my secret was finally leaving my soul for good.

CHAPTER 19
A NEW START

In the days that followed, Liz's campaign was born. We started by setting up a Facebook page called, "Liz Marks" with a profile picture in which we both wore lime-green jackets, chosen by Liz because her car accident scene was documented with lime-green spray paint. We also ordered wristbands in the same color that read "Don't Text N Drive 4 Liz Marks." It was something for her to give to the people she talked to about what had happened to her and why. We felt it could be that "little something" they could take with them as a reminder not to text and drive. I ordered the cheapest and minimum amount of lime-green business cards that I could find online. They contained her campaign slogan and contact information. We handed them out to anyone who was interested in hosting Liz and me to speak about her story.

I started to research whom I could contact to tell her story. I found the websites of three major cell phone companies and emailed them, but they never wrote back. I also found a website called Distracted Driving. GOV, associated with NHTSA (National Highway Traffic Safety Administration), and information for their marketing specialist, Lori Millen. The page included a contact number for people to call in their stories about distracted driving. I called and left a message. The next day, I received a phone call from Lori Millen.

Lori was very open to hearing the story I wanted to tell about Liz and me. After describing Liz's story to Lori, I told her we were in the beginning stages of organizing Liz's campaign to bring awareness to people in the community about the dangers of texting and driving and let her know that we were available as speakers. I could hear the emotion in her voice as she commended us on making the effort to speak about our story and hopefully save lives. We talked on the phone for about 45 minutes, and she ended our conversation by wishing us well in our campaign and telling me that if anything came up, she would be in contact.

The following month, Liz, thanks to her gift of gab, booked several speaking engagements for us. She handed out business cards to anyone who asked for them and brought in engagements that way.

First, we spoke at an after-school program for girls at Tilghman Island Elementary School, which Liz had attended as a child. My palms sweated, and my pulse beat fast like I'd had too much coffee. Liz, on the other hand, remained calm and collected. Girls from 12 to 16 filed into the auditorium. A teacher introduced us, and then we began.

I started by speaking about what parents go through when their child is critically injured in a car accident, and then Liz took over. She showed them pictures of her car accident and pictures of her at the brain rehab center, which really grabbed the girls' attention. She talked about what she had been through and what she was still going through because she chose to text and drive. Our presentation lasted longer than expected due to all the questions the girls had for Liz. I ended the event by playing some music on my totally outdated boom box for the girls to dance to while I videotaped them on my camcorder so they could see themselves on film. We wanted to end the event on a positive note. Liz's story can be overwhelming, and we wanted our audience to leave feeling inspired rather than devastated. We considered the event a success and were able to book another speaking event shortly thereafter.

Next, we rented tables at several craft shows. We divided the table into two sides: one side for the crafts I made to sell to help fund our campaign, the other side for Liz's display about what had happened to her. The lime-green wristbands came in handy; Liz would hold one out to any passerby and use it to hook people into listening to her story. We also spoke at churches, nurses' meetings, Girl Scout meetings, and even set up a table in front of our local grocery store, Food Lion. Word of Liz and her story spread through our town and to its surrounding areas.

One day when we were driving home from a speaking event, Liz was unusually quiet.

"What are you thinking about?" I asked her.

"I think I'd like to make a video about my story and post it on YouTube. I feel like my story is only being heard locally, but people outside of our area need to know about it, too."

"That's a great idea," I said. "We can make the video ourselves."

By making monthly payments, I could afford a newer, more professional video camera with a tripod. First, I called the office of Liz's plastic surgeon, Dr. Dorafshar, and asked his assistant for copies of the pictures taken throughout the stages of Liz's reconstructive surgeries. Within days, we were at his office picking them up. They were graphic and disturbing, but I knew they would be very effective in helping to convey Liz's message.

Next, I called a man by the name of Clay Stamp. I didn't know it at the time, but this phone call would be a big game-changer in the making of Liz's video. The Director of Emergency Services for Talbot County, where Liz had her car accident, he served on the Board of Directors for the Shock Trauma Center in Baltimore. Aware of Liz's accident from reading about it in the local paper, he had come to see her in the ICU, and we had stayed in touch. Now, I needed his help. I wanted recordings of the 911 calls made after Liz's car accident to include in the video we were making.

He listened as I told him how Liz wanted to tell her story through a video with the plan of posting it on YouTube. He asked me who was helping us make this video, and I informed him that we were trying to make this video on our own.

"Hold on," he said. "I think I may know someone who would be interested in helping you with your video."

Mr. Stamp set up a meeting the following week for Liz and me to pitch our story. At the meeting, we spoke to Clay Stamp, a man named Brian LeCates, Deputy Director EMS Chief of Talbot County Department of Emergency Services, and John Gain, Director of Educational Support Services for the Maryland Institute for Emergency Medical Services Systems (MIEMSS).

At the Talbot County 911 Center, Mr. Stamp introduced Liz and me to Mr. Gain and Mr. LeCates, and we went into a meeting room with two tables. The three gentlemen took their seats at one table, and Liz and I set up at the other table across from them. I kept telling the three men to let us know when we should stop, but they kept asking questions and encouraging us to continue. I talked about the day of the accident and showed them the pictures I had obtained from Dr. Dorafshar as well as some pictures of Liz's car accident I had copied from the St. Michaels Fire Department Facebook page.

Liz talked about her many ups and downs during her recovery and how she was admitted to a mental hospital for depression and suicidal thoughts. We wrapped up by telling them about how Liz felt she had lived for a reason—if she shared her story through a video, maybe it would prevent others from making the same grave mistake she had made of texting and driving.

It may sound ridiculous, but we ended our presentation by dancing to the Justin Bieber song *Believe*. We had heard the song on the radio one day while driving, and I felt that the words to this song described what Liz and I had been through over the past year.

All three men were glassy-eyed; it looked like they were trying not to cry. I asked Mr. Stamp if they would help us with our video. He looked at Mr. Gain and Mr. LeCates and then looked back at me.

"Yes."

After saying our goodbyes to the men, Liz and I got in our car. We acted calmly and coolly, but as soon as we knew they were out of earshot, we screamed with joy like two crazy women.

CHAPTER 20

VIRAL

While Liz and I waited for filming of the MIEMSS video to begin, we continued her campaign. Our local newspapers featured articles about Liz and her campaign. We spoke at school prom promise events (a school-hosted event where guest speakers talk about drinking and driving or driving distracted in an effort to keep students safe), driving schools, and even on local TV stations. We spoke at the Fire Department whose volunteers had been dispatched to Liz's car accident, and it was wonderful to have the opportunity to thank the fire fighter volunteers, EMTs, and paramedics who played a part in saving my daughter's life. We also spoke at a ribbon-cutting for a new state-of-the-art helicopter, an emotional event because the medics who had flown Liz to Shock Trauma had been highly instrumental in saving her life. Liz and I also met and became friends with the flight paramedic, Jeremy Krebs, who had kept Liz alive on that flight to the hospital.

Liz still experienced some bad days along with the good days. New medications for her depression caused weight gain, and she became self-conscious not only about her face but also about her body. She had reconnected with Kayla, and they would hang out—but not bowl together; bowling was not Kayla's "thing."

So, Liz spent a lot of time bowling by herself, becoming friends with some of the alley's employees though not with John. Another male employee asked to bowl with her one day, and she readily agreed. When I came to pick her up, she told me they had had a good, friendly time together and it was the first time she had felt normal since her car accident.

When the production of the MIEMSS video finally got off the ground in October 2013, we included as reenactors as many of the original St. Michaels volunteer firefighters, EMTs, and paramedics who were involved in saving Liz's life as possible. We also secured interviews with some of Liz's doctors who performed her lifesaving surgeries, including Dr. Dorafshar. We used the pictures of her mangled car after the accident, but due to legal issues with the original recordings, we were only able to reenact the 911 calls. In the end, Liz and I were very pleased with the video, which ran 11 minutes.

Liz and I decided, however, not to post the video to YouTube because we wanted people, especially students, to see the video for the first time at live events and in Liz's presence. We felt it would have more of an impact to show the video and then have the actual girl in the video come on stage to speak to the audience. This formula proved very effective and evoked a strong emotional response from both students and adults.

Word got around that our presentation was very moving, and before long the requests to speak at high schools came flooding in. A representative for the state of Maryland's Transportation Division also contacted us, and we ended up speaking for a program they sponsored called "Towards Zero Deaths in Maryland." We traveled to many distracted driving events around the state for this program and made our presentation stronger each time we spoke.

I hadn't heard from Lori Millen since our initial conversation about Liz's campaign, but one day in the middle of March 2014, she called me. Lori said that she had never forgotten my daughter's story and wondered if her campaign was ongoing. When I affirmed that it was, she told me that April is National Distracted Driving Awareness Month and the Department of Transportation was having a distracted driving event. Perhaps it would be possible to get Liz and me to come and speak at this event?

Within a week, Liz and I were scheduled to speak at the event and soon after at an event in Washington DC—NHTSA had launched a new campaign against texting and driving called "You Text, You Drive, and You Pay." Before we spoke for NHTSA, we did interviews with TV outlets. Liz did an interview with a Spanish network, and I did an interview with a correspondent from CBS. Unexpectedly, this led CBS's office in DC to invite us to film a segment with their transportation correspondent, Jeff Pegues.

It was a happy, stressful blur, but it represented a major step—CBS and our first national television appearance.

It surprised me again when Lori called a few days later. Her department had received a lot of positive feedback about our appearance and she wanted to know if they could produce a short video about Liz's story, with the intention of posting it to YouTube. It took only a single day to film the short video, at only three minutes long much shorter than the MIEMSS video. A month later, Lori emailed us the final product for our review, and soon thereafter, it went live.

During the first several months, the video received about 30,000 hits, a number that excited Liz and me. Liz monitored our numbers daily; she looked forward to doing that.

On October 29, 2014, right before we had to leave for a scheduled appointment with Dr. Dorafshar, Liz came running into the kitchen and gushed, "My video has 200,000 hits!"

"That's not possible," I said.

"It's true," she said, and opened the computer to show me. When I saw the figure and realized she was right, I felt stunned. I thought to call Lori to see if she might know the reason for the sudden surge, but we didn't have time.

While Liz was being examined by Dr. Dorafshar, she told him the news about her YouTube video, and he looked as stunned as I had. He had his assistant pull up the video on a computer outside his office, and a few minutes later she came in to inform us the video now had 250,000 hits—50,000 more since Liz had checked earlier that morning. Dr. Dorafshar told Liz how proud he was of her and her campaign.

Before we left the hospital, I tried once more to reach Lori. This time, I got through. She investigated and informed me that a woman had shared Liz's video to UPWORTHY.COM, a site with a reputation for posting meaningful stories and reaching a massive audience.

Liz's video was going viral! By the end of that day, the video had received one million hits and continued to climb—a million more the following day and another million over the next two days! Incredible! People from all over the world had requested to be Liz's friend on Facebook. We maxed out at five thousand friends within a day, so we started a public Facebook page called "Don't Text N Drive 4 Liz Marks," which exploded with activity. Liz felt like a celebrity. People posted words of encouragement, shared their own stories about distracted driving, and sent messages about how

Liz's story not only touched them but also scared them. They promised her that they would never use their cell phones behind the wheel again.

It felt both uplifting and sad to see so many people talking about how they could relate to Liz and her feelings of being left out and alone. I let Liz read a few but did not allow her to see them all. So many lonely people poured out their hearts about the emptiness in their lives that I felt it would be too much for Liz. The biggest fear people who had been through accidents like Liz's expressed was dying alone. I tried to message each one back but found myself getting so overwhelmed that I, shamefully, had to stop, unable to respond to them all.

Producers from national television shows started calling. Of those, the daytime show, *The Doctors,* a spin-off of *Dr. Phil,* really excited us. The show features a panel of medical professionals and sometimes celebrity guest speakers, who discuss a variety of health and medical issues. Each doctor weighs in on medical topics, as well as dangers and current events that affect our health. Dr. Travis Stork, an emergency room physician who had appeared on *The Bachelor* in 2012, and Dr. Andrew Ordon, a plastic surgeon, were the co-hosts. Liz and I were going to Hollywood! This would be a great opportunity for Liz and me to thank the medical community for saving her life.

For the next two days, I prepared for the trip, bustling about doing errands and laundry, though secretly feeling anxious. Liz, of course, showed no signs of being nervous and couldn't wait to be on TV.

After Liz's first commercial plane ride, we arrived in Los Angeles, and a car service whisked us to our hotel. The hotel floors gleamed, and the center of the lobby held a park with full-sized trees surrounded by an array of gorgeous, colorful flowers. Neither one of us slept much that night.

We had dressed and descended to the lobby before 8:00 a.m. the next morning, waiting for a producer to come pick us up to take us to the studio. We met another young woman, named Jackie, in the car; she was also taping a segment for *The Doctors* that day. She had a disfiguring medical condition and had used the condition to her advantage, starting a career in modeling. She was a kind, loving person, and meeting her brought us pleasure.

Liz and I had brought our own wardrobes: black pants suits with neon green shirts that represented the color of Liz's campaign, which the producers loved. We had also brought Liz's wristbands.

Hair and makeup experts came to attend to us. Liz was assigned to a lovely woman, with whom she instantly bonded. I could hear them laughing and talking in the next room like old friends.

"You'll be fine; everything is alright," I heard the woman say to Liz, which made me concerned that something was wrong. But when I walked in, Liz turned to face me, and my breath caught in my throat. For the first time since the accident, I could see the old Elizabeth. They had managed to cover most of Liz's scars and had highlighted both of her eyes.

"Look Mom, I'm pretty again," she said. She started to cry.

"If you cry, then all my work will go running down your face," the makeup artist said, and we all started to laugh.

After makeup, we returned to the green room and met with two producers to go over Liz's story and practice answering questions that the hosts might ask us. "If you make a mistake," the producer said, "just correct yourself and move on." Then, we heard a knock on the door.

"Show time."

We entered the studio, which held nearly 100 people, mostly students from a local private high school. We sat upfront with the other guests for the show. It was thrilling to see Dr. Stork and Dr. Ordon, celebrities we'd seen on TV, who were joined by the other two hosts, Dr. James Sears, a pediatrician, and Dr. Rachael Ross, a family physician.

Then came our segment. They showed a portion of Liz's viral video from NHTSA and then panned straight to Liz and me. They spoke to Liz first, and she did an excellent job. Then, they asked me questions. Liz and I talked over Dr. Stork a few times, but he took it in stride. At one point, he put his elbows on the table in front of him and just listened to Liz and me, letting us have the room.

As Dr. Stork wrapped up our segment, I happened to look at Dr. Rachael Ross, and she mouthed to me, "Great job." The segment aired two months later, on January 6, 2015 and was viewed by almost one million people.

CHAPTER 21

MEETING OPRAH

Liz had many more surgeries in her future. Another reconstructive facial procedure was scheduled during the height of our campaign. So, as Liz prepared, underwent the surgery, and then recovered, we put her campaign on temporary hold. The surgery made a noticeable improvement to Liz's facial appearance, another badly needed step toward Liz getting her confidence back. When she went to her post-op appointment, she told Dr. Dorafshar that she wasn't going to have any more work done on her face.

"I'm happy with it," she said. "I don't want to try and make it perfect. It's perfect enough."

"I understand," he said. "I think you are perfect, too. And if you ever change your mind, I will be more than happy to do whatever you want done."

We started to travel regularly nationwide, speaking at school-based distracted driving events, starting with several events in Chicago's inner-city high schools. Since most students there used the city's bus service for transportation, we stressed the importance of not texting and walking. While Liz was at Shock Trauma in Baltimore, I had struck up a conversation with a nurse and asked her which type of accident brings patients to the hospital the most. She surprised me with her answer: "Pedestrian accidents"—more and more people use their cell phones when walking and don't pay attention to where they are going.

~~~~~~~~~~~~~~

Telling her story, especially her mistake, over and over was very hard on Liz. After each event, she would be mentally exhausted: all she wanted to do was get something to eat and go back to the hotel. We hardly did any sightseeing on our extensive American travels.

When we weren't traveling, I tried to make life as normal as possible for Liz. I did not want all the attention to go to her head so I made it a point to keep her grounded. She had chores to do around the house, I gave her an allowance for her fun money, and she was responsible for caring for her dog.

I was also reteaching Liz to drive, a challenge for both of us. What if she gets in another accident? I asked myself constantly, and this concern overshadowed the patience I should have shown her as she was relearning. I wanted her to drive perfectly, an unrealistic goal that only made us both frustrated and argumentative. As the lessons went on, though, we both calmed down, and Liz eventually got her driver's license renewed. Nonetheless, for a long time she did not want to drive on her own. She enjoyed driving but always wanted me to tag along as her security blanket. Eventually, as time passed and she got behind the wheel more often, she embraced driving on her own.

Liz still struggled to make friends. Sure, she had thousands of Facebook friends on both of her pages and was adored by everyone when she spoke, but these were distant friends, strangers really. She did manage to reconnect with one or two of her old friends from high school, girls who had left college and returned home to try to figure out what they wanted to do with their lives. They didn't get together often, but at least it was something. Her uncensored way of speaking, which had offended some of her friends before, was improving, thanks to her cognitive classes and the extensive experience she gained from speaking at events. Her focus had also gotten better so she was able again to watch TV shows and movies.

The only other person with whom Liz would regularly spend time was Jim. Before the car accident, she wanted nothing to do with her stepfather, but afterward, she grew to think of him like a dad. Every Saturday, they went out for breakfast and then shopping. She had him wrapped around her finger and reaped some nice benefits. I had to tell Jim to ease up on spoiling her, but his response was always the same: "If anybody needs a break in life, it's Liz."

After some convincing, Liz got one other thing to make herself feel better—a prosthetic eye. Her blind eye was still intact. She felt no pain and had had no infections so the doctors felt no need to remove the eye. Liz, though, was self-conscious about it. Curious children would ask all the time what had happened to her eye, and she worried what her peers were thinking. Up to this point, though, she had refused to get a prosthetic eye. The complexity of the oculofacial plastic surgery required freaked Liz out. It involved taking out the inner parts of the blind eye and replacing them with a synthetic fill. Then, the inner skin of her eye would be stitched permanently to a closed position to prevent any future infections of the eye area. The procedure would help move her damaged eye position closer to its original position so that she could be fitted for a prosthetic eye shell.

Another angel was sent to help Liz in her recovery period. I had insisted we all join our local YMCA as a family, and one day when Liz was at the YMCA, an older gentleman came up to her and politely asked her about her left eye. After she told him about it, he told Liz that he had lost the sight in one of his eyes while serving in a war. He then asked her to tell him which eye he had lost. She looked straight into his eyes and could not tell which was the blind eye; the two eyes looked exactly the same. He took his finger, raised it up to his right eye, and began to make tapping sounds on his right eyeball.

"But it looks so real!" she exclaimed.

He went on to tell her that his right eye had been removed, and he was wearing a prosthetic eye. After hearing this glowing testament about the benefits of a prosthetic eye, Liz began the long process of getting her own.

The next thing Liz wanted was a hearing aid. She had lost 95 percent of her hearing in her left ear as a result of bones in her ear that had been crushed or broken in the accident. In the coming months, Liz had many appointments with doctors at the Ear, Nose and Throat department of Johns Hopkins to be tested and fitted with her new hearing aid.

~~~~~~~~~~~~~~~

Winter turned to spring. Then, it was April 2015. Liz turned 21, and we celebrated her big day with a dinner at her favorite restaurant, Olive Garden, with family and her good friend, Kayla. The following month, Liz and I started speaking at bigger events and to larger audiences of up to 1,500 people.

We did radio shows, made reappearances on some of our local TV stations, and even presented as keynote speakers at the annual Firemen's Convention in Ocean City, Maryland. After our presentation there, some of the key people involved in saving Liz's life came on stage to surprise Liz and me. They included the state trooper who had made that critical call for the medevac chopper, the nurse who had screamed "Give her the goddam hair," the neurologist who had released Liz's trach tube restraints and witnessed Liz blowing her trach tube across the room, the St Michaels Volunteer Fire Department first responders and medical personnel who had helped to save Liz's life, and the three gentlemen, Clay Stamp, John Gain and Brian LaCates, who had been instrumental in helping us make the MIEMSS video that so greatly enhanced our presentations and warned audience members about the dangers of texting while driving. Needless to say, this was one of our most emotional and memorable speaking events.

Our speaking events continued on strong. Liz's Facebook pages continued to buzz with activity, both with posts of our events and other postings from Facebook friends and followers, as they shared their thoughts and experiences about distracted driving. I would sometimes receive inquiries on these pages from organizations asking how to book us for an upcoming event so I made it a point to be on top of any messages or postings coming to us through these pages.

Then, one day in August 2015, I checked our Facebook pages. I scrolled through the messages—and then saw it: The Holy Grail, the mother lode, the crème de la crème of messages. It read: "Hi Liz, I'm a producer for the Oprah Winfrey Network. Can you please email me your phone number? I'd love to talk to you today if possible. Thanks so much."

I was stunned. Never in my wildest dreams did I think we would ever get a message from Oprah's network. But there it was, clear as day. I had an email and a name to go with it. The first thing I did was hold my phone in the air and shriek, "Oprah Winfrey wants to hear Liz's story!" My heart pounded.

Within minutes, I was talking to this very pleasant woman on the phone. She informed me that she was a follower of Liz's public Facebook page and was amazed by her recovery and all the great work she and I were doing to increase awareness about the dangers of distracted driving. Her boss, Oprah, was a big advocate for educating people about this serious problem. In 2010, on *The Oprah Winfrey Show*, Oprah had aired an episode that focused on the dangers of cell phone use while driving. After her talk show stopped running in 2011, Oprah launched her new show, *Where Are They Now?* on OWN the following year. On this show, Oprah interviewed stars from the worlds of show business, music, and sports, asking them questions about their careers and what they are doing now. Her guests also included people who were not celebrities but had compelling stories to tell. Oprah wanted Liz and me to appear on *Where Are They Now?* She was interested in what Liz had done since the video went viral.

I drove to the shopping center where Liz was hanging out, and when Liz opened the door to my car, I had the biggest grin on my face.

"Why are you smiling?" she asked, suspicious.

"Someone big and important is interested in hearing about your story."

"Ellen?!"

"No, but someone just as big. Oprah."

Her face showed shock and disbelief. "No way."

"Yes way."

The next day Oprah's producer called us back and asked to speak to Liz about her campaign. I handed the phone over and let Liz tell her story. The conversation was on speaker phone so I heard everything and was so proud of Liz and the way she handled herself in that interview.

Later that day, I received the exciting news from the producer that our appearance on the show was approved! We were to fly to LA and meet Oprah in person. We could not tell anyone, though, until after the segment was filmed; after that, we could blab to whomever we wanted.

I asked the producer to tell Liz the great news. I wanted someone other than me to tell her so it would be more exciting. I passed the phone over.

"Liz, you're going to meet Oprah," the producer said.

Liz erupted with howls of joy and excitement.

I took the phone back from Liz. "Sorry for breaking your eardrums," I said.

"It's okay," she said. "Actually, I miss moments like this."

When we entered our room in the Beverly Hills hotel, white robes had been laid on the bed and white slippers on the floor for us to wear. The robes smelled fresh, and the slippers were in a sealed, clear package. Liz ripped open the package, put those puppies on her feet, and wrapped that big, fluffy soft white robe around her body.

We arrived in the afternoon so Liz and I had time to soak in the splendor of Beverly Hills. It was a warm sunny day so we set out on foot. We walked around the area surrounding the hotel and took pictures of everything and anything, just like any typical tourists. The mansions where many of the stars lived were just a couple miles away.

The next morning, bright and early, Liz and I stood in the hotel lobby, waiting to be picked up. A black limo with darkly tinted windows pulled up to the front doors of the hotel, and a man dressed in a black suit, freshly starched white shirt, and shiny, black shoes got out. He entered the lobby, made eye contact with Liz, and asked her if she was Miss Marks.

Liz smiled sweetly. "Yes."

One of Oprah's producers escorted us into the studio, walking us past machines, cameras, and lots of people running around busily. We ended up in a room where makeup artists sat ready to do their magic on us. It was a larger green room than what we had experienced on other shows and was filled with drinks, food, and laughter; everyone seemed at ease with each other. A few people came into the room to introduce themselves to us and thank Liz and me for coming to tell our story.

As the time to film our segment drew near, I could feel myself getting nervous. But Liz had no jitters—she couldn't wait to get out there and meet Oprah. Someone came into the green room and said, "It's time."

We were guided back to the same room that we had passed through before, but this time the room was very dimly lit. The producer told us to watch our steps as we made our way to the center of a small film studio. In the back we saw screens, some with *Where Are They Now?* logos on them, others bearing pictures of Liz, the pictures I had emailed to help tell Liz's story. One picture was a selfie of Liz before the accident. Another was of her car accident scene, and the other screens displayed the pictures that Dr. Dorafshar had taken throughout Liz's recovery stages.

It was then that I noticed three black-leather, high-backed chairs in the middle of this studio room, and on one of those chairs sat Oprah Winfrey. One person at her elbow retouched her makeup while the other went over items on a piece of paper he held in front of her. She wore a lovely, peach-colored blouse with a pair of jeans and fancy high heels. She looked just like she did whenever we watched her on TV—exquisite skin. When we were close enough for the lighting to illuminate us, she made eye contact and in a friendly voice said, "Hello, ladies."

Unlike the studio where *The Doctors* was shot, there was no audience here—just Oprah, Liz, and me. Liz sat down next to Oprah, and I took the other chair. It was a surreal moment.

Once Oprah finished making introductory comments, my nervousness subsided, and the interview proceeded just like any other. When the interview came to an end, out of the corner of my eye, I could see a director signaling for Oprah to wrap it up. She concluded the interview, and then the cameras stopped rolling.

"Good job, ladies," Oprah said. "Good job."

This moment was the highlight of Liz's campaign. It has become a wonderful story to share with our family members, and I know it will be passed down to future generations.

Before we got into the car that would take us back to our hotel, Liz asked the producer if she could post a picture of us with Oprah on her Facebook page. The producer replied that Liz was free to post whatever she wanted. Within seconds, Liz's fingers were working their magic.

CHAPTER 22

THE FUTURE

Even before our segment with Oprah aired, we were getting bombarded with requests to speak from bigger schools and big businesses—Baltimore Gas & Electric and a petroleum refining company in Texas wanted Liz to tell her story to their employees. Our calendar filled up rapidly.

For the next year, Liz and I traveled all over the United States, doing speaking engagements. We went to Johnstown, New York to speak at a high school, Atlanta to speak to the employees of a heating and cooling business, and back to Los Angeles to do a segment on a Hallmark Network show called *Home and Family*. We also had the honor of speaking to the troops at Fort Meade, Maryland and filmed a segment with ABC's show, *Nightline*, at Johns Hopkins Hospital.

With each event, Liz improved her speaking skills. It was amazing to see audiences' reactions to Liz as she walked onstage after the MIEMSS video concluded. You could hear a pin drop; everyone's eyes would be totally glued to Liz as she walked across the stage to reach the podium. In her speeches, Liz talked about feeling ugly and lonely and wanting to hurt herself, but she would always follow up by saying that she was now taking medicine for her depression and sees a therapist to talk about her ups and downs. She told the audiences that she is not a freak; she is a normal person, and seeking help for depression is not shameful. She would encourage anyone experiencing thoughts of wanting to hurt themselves or others please to get help. "I got help, and I just got finished interviewing with Oprah," she would say. "I feel pretty good!"

Once Liz had finished speaking and the applause settled down, she would encourage the audience to ask her questions. Nothing was off limits. If no one was brave enough to raise a hand, I had questions ready like:

- Do you have a boyfriend?
- Are you getting more surgery to your face?
- Do you have brothers or sisters?

Questions like that would get the ball rolling, and sure enough, audience members would start to raise their hands with questions of their own.

Liz would always answer questions completely candidly—she did not hold anything back. She wanted everyone to understand what she had gone through, good and bad, because she had chosen to text and drive. At almost all of her speaking events, people asked questions about her blind eye. She purposely did not wear her prosthetic eye shell when speaking because she wanted everyone to see the damage she had caused herself. When this question came up, Liz would pull the prosthetic eye shell out of her jacket pocket to show the audience who would react with a collective gasp, a very effective technique in getting her point across.

Watching Liz connect with people, especially high school students, was something to behold. I stood back and watched her open her soul to them, hoping to get them to grasp the dangers of distracted driving. But it was more than that; she was also teaching them a life lesson. She was a living example of how unfair life can be and how the way you choose to handle the hard times makes a difference in the way your life turns out. You can play the passive role of victim, or you can seek help and find your purpose. She never imagined that she would be traveling around the country to speak about her story and meeting kind, supportive people along the way.

All the traveling, however, took a toll on Liz and me. We started to argue about trivial things. Then, in January 2017 Liz began saying she wanted to get a normal job, one that didn't require traveling. She felt tired of reliving her story and was not bouncing back after each event as easily as she had before. She still felt lonely; traveling gave her no time to make friends or find a real everyday job. It was time for us to take a break.

It took some time, but Liz landed a part-time job in retail. She also joined a new 24-hour gym, which made it possible for her to work out anytime she wanted. Her doctors stressed to Liz the importance of working out, not only to maintain a healthy weight but also to help with brain recovery. During one of her workouts, Liz met a young man named David. They dated for a while and then broke up. But as often happens with young romance, what was off was soon back on. Only time will tell whether they have a future together. Getting married and one day having children of her own is something Liz sees for herself, but no time soon.

While we greatly appreciate the tireless efforts of all the doctors and medical personnel who treated her, Dr. Dorafshar holds a special place in our hearts. His skill and that of his plastics team have greatly enhanced Liz's quality of life. Dr. Dorafshar's work may not have been the surgery that initially saved her life, but it was the first of many surgeries that would eventually make her happy with the woman she saw in the mirror, scars and all, and which, in turn, gave her the confidence she needed to let go of her old life and embrace her new life.

We saw Dr. Dorafshar for the last time in August 2018 when he told us he was leaving his practice at Johns Hopkins. The reality that he will not be there for us anymore was hard to take in. He referred us to another plastic surgeon he trusted to take over Liz's care and assured us we would be in good hands. We wished him well and told him how much we both would miss him.

Liz still has annual check-ups with her neurologist and also sees him every six months to deal with seizures that she thankfully has under control now. She sees her therapist monthly to help her deal with her ups and downs and her psychiatrist every three months to check on her psychiatric medications. At this time, Liz has no surgeries of any kind in her future, and she couldn't be more thrilled about that.

Liz's physical, cognitive, and depression issues will be something that we as a family will have to deal with for the rest of our lives. She will still have challenges ahead of her from her disabilities, but she is now living the normal life she has so desperately wanted since her car accident. She has new friends. After a six-month break in 2017, she resumed speaking and continues to speak at events here and there. She works part-time at our local grocery store as a cashier and eagerly shares her story with each new person who comes through her line.

~~~~~~~~~~~~~~

As for me, my life is getting back to normal, but it is a new normal. I have learned to live within the moment and fully enjoy the two greatest accomplishments in my life: Logan and Liz. Nothing is more satisfying for a parent than to live long enough to see their children become productive, caring, and well-adjusted adults. For me, being a parent is the hardest but most fulfilling job that I could have, and I truly cherish it.

That it was my text that dramatically altered the course of our lives is something I will never forget. I have forgiven myself, but I will never let it go. I am plagued by it every day, and hope that I have conveyed the message that using your cell phone irresponsibly can have devastating consequences, consequences that can shake your family to its very core.

Through our travels and from the Facebook messages we received, I learned of marriages that have ended due to the financial, physical, and emotional burdens a distracted driving accident had on their relationships. Some families were left completely broke—beyond repair. They lost the family home due to medical bills, the strain that comes with taking care of a disabled loved one became too much, or the loss of a loved one meant living permanently with an empty hole in the heart. These are the families that are in my prayers every night. I pray that they seek help, that they learn to accept their new lives, and that they search for strength and meaning through their God.

As far as our family, we feel blessed beyond measure. So many things had to be in place for Liz to come through her car accident, as well as for her to have no doubt she was saved for a reason. I remember asking God when the accident first happened, Why us? Why Liz? I now know why. It was a path that God chose for us to tread, a journey that almost broke us but that also strengthened us to experience a life that exceeded our plans, expectations, and even dreams. It's an ordeal that I would not wish on anyone but one that I would not take away from my own life. I have experienced life in a way that would never have been possible if I had not gone through hell and back.

Mark Twain said that the two most important days in your life are the day you are born and the day you find out why. It took a near fatal car accident and a chance meeting with a woman at a Walmart for Liz to find out why she was born.

Drive Safely, and Please Pay Attention Behind the Wheel,
Betty Shaw
September 2019

Part Four

DISCUSSION QUESTIONS

Betty Shaw

Here are some questions that can be used by groups, schools, teachers, and others concerned with preventing more deaths from texting and driving:

1) Almost every state in the U.S. has some law in place to penalize distracted drivers, yet people still use their cell phones openly behind the wheel. Why do you think using your cell phone while driving is socially acceptable?

2) According to research conducted by AT&T, 77 percent of American teenagers report adults close to them instruct them not to text and drive, yet they see those same adults texting while driving. How does this make you feel? And are you one of those teens?

3) When Liz was still in ICU, Betty Shaw asked a TRU nurse, "What is the number one reason patients end up in ICU?" Thinking the TRU nurse would say, "Car accidents," Betty was surprised when the nurse responded, "Pedestrian accidents." She said more and more people are using their cell phones while walking and not paying attention to their surroundings. Does this surprise you too?

4) Liz was aware of the dangers of distracted driving before her car accident. Why do you think she chose to ignore the warnings?

5) The book addresses how Liz felt tremendous guilt for causing so much worry and pain to her family and friends. How did this affect her recovery?

6) In the beginning stages of Liz's recovery, she expressed herself exactly as she felt; she had no filter. How did this impact her relationships with her friends and family?

7 Liz's mother ignored the cognitive therapist's advice to seek professional mental help for her daughter due to the stigma associated with mental illness. Do you feel this stigma is just?

8) What can we do as a society to alleviate the negative mindset about people getting help for mental health issues?

9) Mass shootings have more than doubled since Columbine and now occur with alarming frequency. Is this due to mentally ill people not undergoing treatment for their disease, the lack of gun control in our country, or both?

10) In the book, Betty Shaw describes the many Facebook messages from people who could relate to Liz and her feelings of loneliness and being left out. What can you do to help someone you know who has these same feelings?

11) In view of what you've read about our family's crash, what are you doing to stop distracted driving by your family? Start with yourself—are you setting a good example?

12) In the event of a crash (and it doesn't have to be catastrophic as our family's), are you prepared to cover the potential costs? Here are some of the issues you need to consider:

   a) Do you have good health insurance, and does it cover long-term care or catastrophic injuries?

   b) Could a parent afford to take a leave of absence to care for an injured family member?

   c) Could you afford to pay for repairs or buy another car?

   d) Could you afford to pay an attorney's fees to defend a lawsuit for punitive damages if the crash was caused by you or a family member?

13) Now consider the emotional toll of a distracted driving accident. If your family has to change its entire lifestyle, how would the dynamics of your family be affected? Could your family survive emotionally?

14) What if you and/or your child caused somebody's death because of distracted driving? Would you and/or your child be able to handle experiencing the grief associated with knowing it was your fault? How do you think you or your child would be treated by friends and associates?

Distracted driving accidents cause what we call a "ripple effect" because the crash doesn't just happen in a vacuum, but instead the ripples continue to spread.

Thanks to Lori Miller of USDOT for her contribution to this section.

STATISTICS

Distracted Driving claimed 3,166 lives in 2017. Source: NHTSA

Distracted Driving now kills more teenagers than alcohol. Source: TeenSafe

2.35 million people in the U.S. are injured or disabled by car crashes every year. More than 330,000 of these crashes that result in severe injury are caused by texting and driving. Source: TeenSafe

For the past decade, distracted driving has taken U.S. roadways by storm, endangering not only distracted drivers but also their passengers, people in other vehicles, and pedestrians. Source: NHTSA

RESOURCES

Distracted Driving/NHTSA (https://www.nhtsa.gov)

TeenSafe (http://teensafe.com)

SELECT MSI BOOKS

Health & Fitness

108 Yoga and Self-Care Practices for Busy Mommas (Gentile)

Girl, You Got This! (Renz)

Living Well with Chronic Illness (Charnas)

Survival of the Caregiver (Snyder)

The Optimistic Food Addict (Fisanick)

Memoirs

57 Steps to Paradise: Finding Love in Midlife and Beyond (Lorenz)

Blest Atheist (Mahlou)

Building a Life from Foreign Parts (Leaver)

Forget the Goal, the Journey Counts . . . 71 Jobs Later (Stites)

From Deep Within: A Forensic and Clinical Psychologist's Journey (Lewis)

One Family: Indivisible (Greenebaum)

Good Blood: A Journey of Healing (Schaffer)

Healing from Incest: Intimate Conversations with My Therapist (Henderson & Emerton)

It Only Hurts When I Can't Run: One Girl's Story (Parker)

Las Historias de Mi Vida (Ustman)

Of God, Rattlesnakes, and Okra (Easterling)

Travels with Elly (MacDonald)

Tucker and Me (Harvey)

Psychology & Philosophy

Anger Anonymous: The Big Book on Anger Addiction (Ortman)

Anxiety Anonymous: The Big Book on Anxiety Addiction (Ortman)

Awesome Couple Communication (Pickett)

Depression Anonymous: The Big Book on Depression Addiction (Ortman)

El Poder de lo Transpersonal (Ustman)

How to Live from Your Heart (Hucknall)

Noah's New Puppy (Rive with Henderson) [PTSD]

Road Map to Power (Husain & Husain)

The Marriage Whisperer: How to Improve Your Relationship Overnight (Pickett)

The Power of Grief (Potter)

The Rose and the Sword: How to Balance Your Feminine and Masculine Energies (Bach & Hucknall)

The Seven Wisdoms of Life (Tubali)

Understanding the Analyst: Socionics in Everyday Life (Quinelle)

Understanding the Critic: Socionics in Everyday Life (Quinelle)

Understanding the Entrepreneur: Socionics in Everyday Life (Quinelle)

Understanding the People around You: An Introduction to Socionics (Filatova)

Understanding the Seeker: Socionics in Everyday Life (Quinelle)

Self-Help Books

100 Tips and Tools for Managing Chronic Illness (Charnas)

A Woman's Guide to Self-Nurturing (Romer)

Creative Aging: A Baby Boomer's Guide to Successful Living (Vassiliadis & Romer)

Divorced! Survival Techniques for Singles over Forty (Romer)

Helping the Disabled Veteran (Romer)

How to Get Happy and Stay That Way: Practical Techniques for Putting Joy into Your Life (Romer)

How to Live from Your Heart (Hucknall) (Book of the Year Finalist)

Life after Losing a Child (Young & Romer)

Publishing for Smarties: Finding a Publisher (Ham)

Recovering from Domestic Violence, Abuse, and Stalking (Romer)

RV Oopsies (MacDonald)*The Widower's Guide to a New Life* (Romer) (Book of the Year Finalist)

Widow: A Survival Guide for the First Year (Romer)

Widow: How to Survive (and Thrive!) in Your 2d, 3d, and 4th Years (Romer)

CPSIA information can be obtained
at www.ICGtesting.com
Printed in the USA
BVHW041113031019
560095BV00004BA/5/P

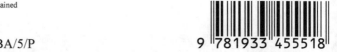